How Is
Get Skinny the Smart Way
Different?

This is not a one-size-fits-all diet, but a customized approach to eating that caters to your individual tastes and preferences—and includes *no* "off-limits" foods.

More than just a food plan, this is a total, active lifestyle program that puts old habits to rest—and rewards you instantly with the benefits of looking and feeling your best.

Here are countless secrets to success—and tips on developing your personalized exercise plan, powerful dieting aids, portion control, and much more.

After reading GET SKINNY THE SMART WAY, you'll never think of "diet" as a four-letter word again.

Books by Annette B. Natow and Jo-Ann Heslin

The Antioxidant Vitamin Counter

Calcium Counts

Count On a Healthy Pregnancy

The Calorie Counter (Second Edition)

The Carbohydrate, Sugar and Fiber Counter

The Cholesterol Counter (Fifth Edition)

The Diabetes Carbohydrate and Calorie Counter

Eating Out Food Counter

The Fat Attack Plan

The Fat Counter (Fifth Edition)

The Food Shopping Counter

Get Skinny the Smart Way

Megadoses

The Most Complete Food Counter

No-Nonsense Nutrition for Kids

The Pocket Encyclopedia of Nutrition

The Pocket Fat Counter (Second Edition)

The Pocket Protein Counter

The Pregnancy Nutrition Counter

The Protein Counter

The Sodium Counter

Published by POCKET BOOKS

Get Skinny the Smart Way

Your Personalized Weight Attack Plan

Annette B. Natow, Ph.D., R.D.
and Jo-Ann Heslin, M.A., R.D.

Illustrations by
Vickie Kalajian Heit

POCKET BOOKS
New York   London   Toronto   Sydney   Singapore

An *Original* Publication of POCKET BOOKS

 POCKET BOOKS, a division of Simon & Schuster, Inc.
1230 Avenue of the Americas, New York, NY 10020

Copyright © 2002 by Annette B. Natow and Jo-Ann Heslin

ISBN: 0-7434-1827-1

First Pocket Books trade paperback printing January 2002

10 9 8 7 6 5 4 3 2 1

POCKET and colophon are registered trademarks of Simon & Schuster, Inc.

For information regarding special discounts for bulk purchases,
please contact Simon & Schuster Special Sales at 1-800-456-6798
or business@simonandschuster.com

Cover design by John Vairo, Jr.

Printed in the U.S.A.

To our families, who support us throughout every project:

Harry, Allen, Irene, Sarah, Meryl,
Laura, Marty, George, Emily, Steven,
Joe, Kristen, Brian and Karen.

Acknowledgments

For graciously sharing their knowledge: Martin Lefkowitz, M.D. and Irene E. Rosenberg, M.D.

For helping us set up the activity and exercise sections of *Get Skinny the Smart Way:* Kathleen Citarrella, M.S., P.T., physical therapist, ProFit Orthopedic and Sports Physical Therapy, New York, and Karen J. Heslin, M.Ed., exercise physiologist, University of Toledo.

For reading the book in its many stages of progress: Jonesie Clemence, Arnie Lubitz, Florence Lubitz, Barbara Natow, John Nolan, and Kristen Robinson.

For all her support and help, our agent, Nancy Trichter.

Without the tireless cooperation of Steven Natow, M.D., and Stephen Llano, *Get Skinny the Smart Way* would never have been completed.

And, a special thank you to our editor, Amanda Ayers, and to everyone who has asked us questions, over the years, about how to successfully lose weight and maintain weight loss. You've taught us a great deal.

"The time to adjust the diet is when the tendency to store fat begins to appear."

". . . it would be better for sedentary people to take some vigorous exercise for their general health. This is particularly true of brain workers and all whose work involves nervous rather than muscular tension."

—Mary Swartz Rose, Ph.D.
Feeding the Family,
The Macmillan Company, 1919

Contents

Preface

Ten years ago we wrote *The Fat Attack Plan*, a successful diet and health plan that over 250,000 readers used to achieve their goal of being slimmer and healthier. What we wrote 10 years ago, in principle, is still accurate and the eating plan is effective. But we wouldn't recommend it to you today.

An accurate and effective way to lose weight and be healthier and yet the experts who wrote it don't recommend it? Sounds crazy, you say. The principles of healthy eating and effective weight loss haven't changed in the last 10 years but the environment in which we buy food, eat, work and play has changed dramatically. Ten years ago, there were few if any lowfat and nonfat foods on the market. Fat substitutes, like Olestra, had not yet been approved. Portions were more reasonable. Bagels didn't weigh 6 ounces. Beverage refills weren't limitless. And restaurant dinner plates were almost 3 inches smaller.

In the past decade the proliferation of new foods has been mind-boggling. The lowfat/nonfat food category has exploded. You can even buy lowfat pet food today. New snack products, cookies, candies and drinks have burst onto the scene offering endless varieties and endless temptation. Everything has gotten bigger. "Big Gulp," "Value-Sized," and "Grande" are the norm. It is impossible to find a "small" in any food category. Add to this our busy lives and jobs that have most of us sitting all day. Life has truly changed in the twenty-first century.

Advice on how to eat today must not only take into account the basic principles of good eating, but it also has to consider the marketplace and lifestyle in which we live. *Get Skinny the Smart Way: Your Personalized Weight Attack Plan* does that and more.

Chapter 1

What the Experts Are Saying

Sixty-one percent of adults are overweight or obese.
Normal weight people are now in the minority.

—Eileen Kennedy, D.Sc., R.D.,
former Deputy Undersecretary, USDA

"Weighing too much can kill you."

Being overweight shortens your life. Excess body fat puts you at higher risk for premature death, even if you are healthy and don't smoke. It's been estimated that obesity causes 300,000 premature deaths a year in this country. In a study of more than one million people, conducted by the American Cancer Society, there were many more deaths among those who were overweight in every age group. This connection was especially significant in the over-75 age group.

"Weighing too much will make you sick."

Weighing too much puts you at risk for heart disease, diabetes, stroke, high blood pressure, arthritis, gout, sleep apnea (disturbed breathing), gallstones, depression, high cholesterol and high blood sugar. Obesity is responsible for 19% of all heart disease, 57% of adult-onset diabetes, 30% of gallbladder disease, 10% of muscle and bone disease, and slightly over 2% of all cancers. Significantly overweight women are more than twice as likely to die from breast cancer as women of normal weight.

Carrying around too many extra pounds stresses the joints, causing aches and pains and a lowered energy level. Less activity can, in itself, lead to further weight gain. As weight climbs, so does blood pressure, cholesterol, triglycerides and blood sugar levels. Higher levels of all of these are predictors of serious health problems and possible illness.

Researchers at Boston University and at the California Birth Defects Monitoring Program found that very overweight women were at least twice as likely as thinner women to have babies with serious birth defects. These findings are significant when you realize that 10% of all women of childbearing age are too heavy.

SMART STUFF

Many overweight women believe gaining weight at menopause can't be avoided. Data from the Massachusetts Women's Health Study showed this is not true. The study found that neither menopause nor the use of hormone replacement therapy was related to weight gain.

"Overweight costs billions."

Two Harvard researchers, Anne Wolf and Graham Colditz, have estimated the annual U.S. bill for obesity at almost $70 billion. The researchers further estimate that an additional $23 billion is spent yearly on indirect costs related to being significantly overweight, such as lost productivity and lost earnings due to hospital stays and early death. Obesity is responsible for over 9% of our national health care costs. Over and above this, the American Dietetics Association estimates that Americans spend another $33 billion a year on products to lose weight.

"Overweight people face discrimination daily."

Overweight people deal with negative reactions on a daily basis. Airline seats, restaurant booths, turnstiles, revolving doors, phone booths, even department store dressing rooms are made with average-size people in mind. When you are larger than average, daily activities are not only difficult but often embarrassing.

Appearance is important. Large people have less choices when it comes to stylish clothes. Employers may be reluctant to put overweight employees in public positions, worrying about the company's perceived image. Employers also worry that overweight employees may create insurance liabilities by taking more sick days because of illness and accidents.

Though state and federal laws forbid discrimination against women, minorities, older workers and the handicapped, there is little or no protection against weight discrimination. Even with unemployment at its lowest level in 30 years, significantly overweight people face discrimination, no matter how qualified they may be, on the job and when looking for a new job.

Company recruiters who say their companies have policies against job discrimination will admit, off the record, that an applicant's weight does matter. Mark V. Roehling, Associate Professor at the Haworth College of Business at Western Michigan University, says, "Employers are more likely to discriminate against people because of their weight than because of their sex or their race."

"The U.S. population is getting fatter every year."

On any given day, 45% of women and 24% of men in the U.S. are either trying to lose weight or maintain the weight they've lost. Another 28% are trying not to gain any additional weight. That leaves very few adults who are not thinking about their weight on a daily basis.

In 1991, one out of eight adults was overweight. By 1998, the statistic had risen to one in five! The National Center for Health Statistics shows that the average American woman age 20 and over is 5 feet, 4 inches, and weighs 152 pounds; the average man over age 20 is 5 feet, 9 inches and weighs 180 pounds. Some of our clients claim their weight problem is due to their genes. Experts from the Centers for Disease Control and Prevention (CPC) do not agree. They point to the startling rise in obesity between 1991 and 1999 but stress that this is far too short a time span for the evolutionary process to significantly change the gene pool in the U.S.

In 1999, 61% of all American adults were overweight; 22% were significantly overweight, with an almost 6% increase in this very overweight group occurring in just one year. In contrast, the 1994 National Health and Nutrition Examination Surveys (NHANES) showed that few adults were significantly overweight in the late 1970s. The next NHANES survey, covering the early 1990s, showed the percentage of significantly overweight adults rose. During the years 1991 through 1999 there was a nearly 60% increase in the number of significantly overweight adults in the U.S.!

The actual number of overweight people in this country may be even larger than estimated because when asked to self-report, people tend to overestimate their height and underestimate their weight. Experts predict that if the nation's weight gain trend continues, in the not-too-distant future, *all* adults in America will be overweight!

SMART STUFF

Sadly, 25% of children in this country are overweight, and the trend shows no sign of reversing.

"A Body Mass Index (BMI) below 25 is healthy."

Overweight is defined as 10 to 20% above your target weight with a BMI (Body Mass Index) between 25 to 30. Obesity (significant overweight) is 30 pounds or more above your target weight with a BMI of 30 or more. A recent national survey reported one third of U.S. adults have a BMI of 29 or higher! According to researchers at the University of Glasgow in Scotland, high BMIs create difficulty with daily activities like bending, kneeling and climbing stairs.

Body mass index (BMI) is a mathematical formula that arrives at a number based on a person's height and weight. You'll determine your BMI in Chapter 7. In 1998, the National Heart, Lung and

Blood Institute (NHLBI) lowered the body mass index number that is the dividing line between average weight and overweight. A BMI between 18.5 and 24.9 is considered healthy. Those with a BMI of 25 and higher are considered to be overweight. Many studies have shown a BMI over 30 increases the risk for death from 50 to 150%.

Among healthy, nonsmoking white men and women and black men, a gradually increasing risk of death begins with a BMI of 25. That translates into 150 pounds for a 5 foot, 5 inch woman, and 175 pounds for a 5 foot, 10 inch man. When the BMI reaches 40 or more, white men are more than two and half times more likely to die; white women twice as likely to die. Surprisingly, black women do not face this increased risk of death, even when they are very overweight.

"Regular physical activity and weight control is a national priority."

Looking to food as a preventive health measure is a recent concept in American public health policy. It started with the 1977 publication of *Dietary Goals for the United States* by the Senate Select Committee on Nutrition and Human Needs. It was the first major step toward the development of a national nutrition health policy and set in motion the development of the first edition of *Dietary Guidelines for Americans,* released in 1980 as a joint effort by the U.S. Department of Agriculture (USDA) and the Department of Health and Human Services (DHHS).

The dietary guidelines help people to make food choices and are based on current research information. To stay up-to-date with scientific developments, they have been revised every five years and since 1990 the federal government has required this periodic review. The latest revision, published in 2000, increased the guidelines from seven to ten healthy principles.

The first and second guidelines are:

1. Aim for a healthy weight.
2. Be physically active each day.

Healthy People 2010, a national health assessment plan developed by the DHHS, prioritizes 28 leading health indicators that need to be moved in a more positive direction to ensure the health of Americans. Two of the most important priorities are:

1. Increase the number of adults who engage in 30 minutes of moderate physical activity every day from 15% of the people to 30%.
2. Reduce the number of adults who are obese from 23% of the population to 15%.

The American College of Sports Medicine (ACSM), the Centers for Disease Control and Prevention (CDC), the American Heart Association (AHA), the National Institutes of Health (NIH), and the President's Council on Physical Fitness and Sports have all recently issued recommendations for regular, moderate intensity, physical activity for everyone. To quote former Surgeon General C. Everett Koop, "It's time to get off your seat and on your feet." Sadly, few are heeding this advice.

SMART STUFF—Put down the remote!
The average American spends 23 hours a week watching TV, equal to one day a week or 10 years over a lifetime!

Over 60% of Americans get no regular exercise and 25% are full-time couch potatoes. TV watching, surfing the Net, electronic games and unsafe streets limit activity. As a country, we move less. Our economy has seen a shift from manufacturing to service industries where most jobs require little physical activity. We drive instead of walk, take elevators instead of stairs, and machines now wash clothes, mow grass and even brush our teeth for us.

"Fat consumption appears to be declining but weight continues to rise."

According to USDA statistics, the average daily calorie intake has increased from 1,854 to 2,002 over the last 20 years. It's been reported, over and over, that fat intake has declined in the last decade, from 37% to 34% of total calories a day. This percentage decrease is misleading. As calories eaten each day have gone up, the actual amount of fat eaten (about 80 grams) has remained fairly constant. When people are eating more calories each day, the percentage of fat calories (out of total calories) will show a decline.

SMART STUFF

More people wear gym clothes than go to the gym!

The Sporting Goods Manufacturers' Association reported that the U.S. consumer spent $286 million on active wear in 1995. Athletic shoes made up for the biggest boost in sales. Since 1992 the sales of hiking/outdoor shoes have tripled, the sales of walking shoes have doubled, and the sales of cross-training athletic shoes rose 32%. It makes you wonder what all those shoes are being used for!

Over the last decade the American public has been bombarded with messages that foods high in fat—like steaks, whole milk, butter and ice cream—put on pounds while food without fat doesn't. The truth is that foods high in fat are more calorie dense. But all foods have calories. It's the portion size that's the problem. As a nation we are convinced that lowfat and nonfat foods have no limits. We can eat what we want, as much as we want, whenever we want, as long as the food is fat free. We are devouring boxes of fat free cookies and slathering nonfat dressing on salads. The calorie excesses from these reduced fat foods are taking their toll and many brands, once touted as the dieters' windfall, have become their downfall.

"People talk a good diet but that's not what they eat."

Have you ever met a person who admitted to raiding the refrigerator in the middle of the night, eating a whole bag of potato chips or keeping candy in their desk drawer? When asked, most sound like health fanatics, munching on rice cakes and sipping water after a 5-mile morning run!

Government researchers have the same problem getting truthful and accurate answers on food surveys. Sometimes people are embarrassed to report what they've eaten because they realize their choices were not the best. Often people can't accurately estimate the amount of food they've eaten. Regardless of the reason, researchers are aware that most people underreport less desirable food items and overreport the healthier ones. And in all cases, people have difficulty estimating amounts.

"People are unable to accurately estimate how much they eat."

A research trend that has held steady over time is the consistent observation that people have more difficulty estimating portion sizes as the size of the portion increases. "Typical" portions in the U.S. are getting bigger and bigger: many restaurants give unlimited beverage, bread, and side dish refills; pasta portions are enormous; bagels resemble frisbees; and a medium-size movie theater popcorn at 16 cups is 13 cups larger than a medium portion in 1957.

Another distinct trend is that people who usually eat smaller portions tend to overestimate their size, whereas those who eat larger portions routinely underestimate them. Studies that have compared the ability of overweight and normal-weight people to estimate portion sizes have reported no difference. Overall, the evidence suggests that difficulties estimating portion size are common across all weight categories and among all age groups.

"When it comes to healthy eating, people aren't sure who to believe."

Americans are bombarded with advice about choosing healthy foods. Most daily newspapers have a regular food section; TV and radio news is full of the findings from the latest scientific studies; whole magazines are devoted to fitness and healthy eating; and store shelves are loaded with the latest dieting gimmicks. And if that isn't enough to sort through, the advice is continually changing. When surveyed, three out of four Americans believe there is too much conflicting information about what to eat.

Eat less fat because fat makes you fat. Eat less carbohydrates because they make you insulin resistant and lead to weight gain. Eat more protein because protein makes you feel full and helps the pounds melt away. Add to that the weight control supplements that suggest you can lose weight in your sleep and the diet drinks that guarantee success in a can and it's no wonder people are confused.

End the Confusion, Get the Facts Straight

Get Skinny the Smart Way will sort out this confusion once and for all.

First—*anything that sounds too good to be true, probably is.*

>*Get Skinny the Smart Way* makes no magic promises except to promise that if you follow our advice you will lose weight.

Second—*anything that promises instant results with little or no effort, won't deliver.*

>*Get Skinny the Smart Way* can't guarantee that you will lose 15 pounds in 5 days. But if you stay with the diet and incorporate its tips and tricks into your daily behavior, you'll not only reach your target weight but you'll hold onto it for the rest of your life.

Third—*be sure the weight loss plan you select is based on well-documented research, not anecdotes from a few success stories.*

>*Get Skinny the Smart Way* is based on years of evolving research about how to lose weight and keep it off. As food professionals with graduate degrees and years of experience, our job is to act as your translator. We take the most current scientific evidence available and turn it into the choices on your dinner plate. The extensive bibliography at the back of the book is the evidence. We invite you to explore it further.

Fourth—*make sure the weight loss plan is tailor-made to your needs and your goals, not a one-size-fits-all diet.*

>*Get Skinny the Smart Way* guides you, through a careful examination of your history, toward setting up future target goals for weight, health and exercise that are designed for you and only you.

Last, and most important—*a diet must assure you that you'll lose weight without causing damage to your health.*

Get Skinny the Smart Way is a *diet that does no harm.* You can be assured of that. We have seen, firsthand, the devastating effects suffered by people who lost their health in the quest for a slimmer body. As dietitians and nutritionists, we have spent our professional careers helping people to live healthier through food. We want to help you.

Chapter 2

More Trips to the Doctor

Currently, obesity-related healthcare costs between $60 and $70 billion a year.

—Centers for Disease Control and Prevention

Weighing Too Much Causes Illness

Simply being overweight puts you at risk for health problems. Five of the ten leading causes of death in the U.S.—heart disease, cancer, diabetes, stroke and atherosclerosis (hardening of the arteries)—are linked to being overweight.

Women in the Nurses' Health Study and men in the Health Professionals' Follow-up Study, who kept their weight within 4 pounds of what they weighed when they were 18 to 20 years old, were healthier than subjects who gained 11 to 22 pounds. Research subjects who put on extra pounds have a 1.5 to 3 times greater risk of heart disease, high blood pressure, gallstones and type 2 diabetes than those who stay slim. As weight goes up, so does risk.

People who are significantly overweight (obese) have an even greater than average risk for serious health problems. They also have a higher incidence of high cholesterol, high triglycerides, stroke, sleep apnea and other breathing problems, arthritis, gout, some cancers, and reduced fertility. More than 70% of significantly overweight people have at least one serious health problem.

SMART STUFF

Weight reduction of as little as 5 to 10% can substantially lower blood pressure, cholesterol, triglycerides, and blood sugar levels.

Heart Disease

Heart disease is America's number one killer. That's the bad news, but the good news is that many deaths can be prevented. The American Heart Association has classified obesity, by itself, as a major risk. Additionally, being overweight worsens other serious risks for heart disease—high blood pressure, high cholesterol, high triglycerides, and insulin resistance, which can lead to diabetes.

Having too much fat around the belly is a risk factor for heart disease. But this fat is very active, which is good. With as little as a 5 to 10% weight loss, more fat is lost from the belly than from other areas of the body. The risk for heart disease goes down as the belly gets smaller.

A study in the *International Journal of Obesity* showed that when a group of significantly overweight people lost weight, their cholesterol, blood pressure, and blood sugar levels went down. Losing weight reduced the risk for heart attack, stroke, and diabetes.

SMART STUFF

For adults, a waist size of more than 35 inches for women, and more than 40 inches for men are signs of extra belly fat, increasing the risk for heart disease and other serious health problems.

Buildup of plaque in the arteries can interfere with blood circulation and this starts early. Autopsies on people who died as early as ages 30 to 34 showed that 20% percent of the men and 8% of the women had plaque narrowing their arteries. The rate of plaque buildup in the arteries was three times higher in overweight people than in leaner people. When people lose weight, the rate of clogging of the carotid artery in the neck slows down. This greatly reduces their risk of a stroke.

In a study in the *Journal of the American Medical Association,* Ming Wei, M.D. and associates in Dallas, Texas found that low cardiorespiratory (heart and breathing) fitness was a strong, independent predictor of heart disease. It was as important a risk as diabetes and smoking. In Dr. Wei's study, subjects were followed for almost ten years. Subjects with low cardiorespiratory fitness were more likely to die. Based on these findings, the researchers recommended that all overweight and significantly overweight people be tested for their level of fitness. At the very least, doctors should be encouraged to do physical activity evaluations on all their overweight patients.

SMART STUFF

There are more heart attacks during the holiday season than at any other time of the year. Too much food and alcohol, as well as increased stress, are believed to be the reasons for the heart attack peak from Thanksgiving to the New Year.

High Blood Cholesterol

Forty years ago cholesterol levels were considered normal at 300 milligrams or less. Back then it wasn't an important medical issue. Today, Americans are encouraged to keep their cholesterol below 200 milligrams. The Framingham Heart study, started by the National Heart, Lung and Blood Institute (NHLBI) in 1955, was the research that made Americans more aware of the importance of their cholesterol number.

Results from this ongoing study showed that as cholesterol levels went up, the risk for a heart attack went up as well. Many other studies, done after the Framingham study, confirmed these findings. Reducing high cholesterol reduces the risk of heart attack and death. Losing as little as 10% of body weight lowers cholesterol and reduces the risk of heart disease by 20%.

SMART STUFF

Studies show that high blood pressure and breathing disorders during sleep are related to each other and both are caused by being overweight.

High Blood Pressure (Hypertension)

One third of all cases of high blood pressure in the U.S. are caused by being significantly overweight. In men under age 45, 60% of those who are overweight also have high blood pressure. Losing weight reduces your blood pressure.

In the Framingham Heart Study, men who lost 15% of their weight had a 10% drop in one measure of their blood pressure. Other studies showed even greater improvement in significantly overweight people who were able to maintain a 10 to 20% weight loss over three years.

Weight training lowers risks for heart disease. The American Heart Association reported that people who lifted weights had a 2% reduction in systolic blood pressure (pressure while the heart is beating) and a 4% reduction in diastolic pressure (pressure while the heart is resting). This may not seem like much, but it could make the difference between a diagnosis of high blood pressure and one of normal blood pressure.

SMART STUFF—Take the stairs

Burning as few as 150 calories a day through activity reduces the risk of high blood pressure, heart disease, diabetes and cancer.

Diabetes

Almost 6% of the population, or 16 million Americans, have diabetes. Another 6 million have it but don't know it. Between 1991 and 1999, there was a 33% increase in new cases of diabetes. The number is expected to rise to 22 million by 2025.

Diabetes can be the direct result of getting too little activity and being too heavy, particularly if most of your weight is around the belly. Even small weight losses, as little as 10 pounds, and a minimal increase in activity improve diabetes control.

Diabetes is a major cause of blindness, kidney failure and leg amputations. It dramatically increases a person's risk of heart disease and stroke. Each year 80,000 Americans die from diabetes and the complications it causes. There are two main types: type 1 and type 2. In both, there is an abnormally high, unhealthy buildup of sugar (glucose) in the blood because the body cannot use this source of fuel.

Type 2 diabetes accounts for 90 to 95% of all cases. Type 2 used to be called adult-onset diabetes because it usually appeared after age 40. Today, as people are getting heavier, more and more younger people are developing type 2 diabetes. It is no longer a disease seen in middle-aged and older people. In the last 10 years, diabetes has risen 70% among those in their thirties. More than 80% of those with type 2 diabetes are overweight. Being slightly overweight increases a person's risk 2 times; being significantly overweight increases the risk for diabetes 10 times.

Cancer

People who are physically active and maintain a healthy weight are less likely to develop colon cancer according to research done at the University of Arizona. People in this study who exercised daily—a 30-minute jog or 60-minute walk—had reduced levels of a hormone-like substance associated with colon cancer. The researchers concluded that when the body mass index (BMI) goes up, so does the risk of colon cancer.

Accumulating evidence shows that being significantly over-weight increases the risk for breast, endometrial (lining of the uterus), cervical, ovarian, gallbladder, colon and prostate cancer.

Adults who gain more than 12 pounds seem to be at greater risk of developing growths (polyps) in the colon and rectum, which can be precancerous. In a 12-year long study of cancer patients by the American Cancer Society, overweight men had a higher rate of colon, rectal, and prostate cancer than lean men. There was a 50 to 70% greater risk of developing colon cancer in overweight men. The risk was particularly strong among older men who were significantly overweight.

Overweight men also have a greater risk for cancer of the kidney. Researchers from the National Cancer Institute and the Umea University in Sweden found that men with the highest body mass index (BMI) were at twice the risk of men with the lowest BMI.

Overweight women have higher rates of some cancers, including breast cancer. Harvard researchers found that women who gained 44 to 55 pounds after age 18 had a 40% higher risk of developing breast cancer after menopause than women who remained slim. Postmenopausal women who are significantly overweight have a greater risk of breast cancer and are more than twice as likely to die from it than normal weight women.

Being significantly overweight, especially from weight gained later in life, increases a woman's risk of developing cancer of the uterus. A study at the Fred Hutchinson Cancer Research Center in Seattle compared the weight of women with and without uterine cancer. Women with uterine cancer were almost three times more likely to be significantly overweight and diabetic than the cancer-free women. In other words, maintaining a healthy body weight and staying physically active can reduce a woman's risk of uterine cancer.

As being overweight becomes more common, the incidence of some forms of throat and stomach cancer are increasing. A Swedish study compared cancer sufferers with healthy people. Those with a body mass index (BMI) higher than 30 were 16 times more likely to develop esophageal (throat) cancer than thinner subjects.

SMART STUFF

A study in the *Journal of the National Cancer Institute* found that men with waists larger than 36 inches and women with waists larger than 32 inches had twice the risk of colon and rectal cancer than people with smaller waists.

Overweight people may have a weaker immune system than normal weight people. The immune system is the body's natural defense against infection or disease. Researchers at Appalachian State and Loma Linda universities studied women, aged 25 to 75, who were mildly to significantly overweight compared to normal weight women of the same ages. They found that increased weight caused several body changes that reduced immune function and increased the risk for cancer. Being significantly overweight increases the levels of growth hormones that encourage the reproduction of cancerous cells. Diets high in calories, sugar and fat, may stimulate tumor growth. In contrast, regular physical activity appears to discourage cancer cell growth in some organs.

If You're Still Not Convinced, There's More . . .

Gallstones—occur 3 to 6 times more often in overweight people; 70% of all gallstones occur in significantly overweight women.

Arthritis—or inflamed joints, are increasing in the U.S., affecting 12% of all adults. Overweight people are 6 times more likely to have arthritis of the knee.

Gout—is a condition caused by uric acid deposits in body tissues and joints, causing inflammation and pain. Significantly overweight people have higher levels of uric acid in their blood.

Sleep—in adequate amounts is vital for good health. People who are significantly overweight sleep less at night and more during the day—dozing and napping. It has been shown that people who are sleep deprived are less active and eat more, increasing the risk of becoming obese.

Cataracts—are the leading cause of blindness world-wide. A body mass index (BMI) higher than 27.8 and fat around the waist are both risk factors for cataracts.

Liver Disease—can lead to cirrhosis and liver failure. Significantly overweight people have a greater risk of liver disease.

It's pretty clear that being too heavy puts you at risk for serious health problems. But enough bad news, let's talk about good news instead. *Get Skinny the Smart Way* can help you lose those extra pounds. You'll be slimmer, feel better, look better, be healthier and live longer. It's worth the effort.

Chapter 3

It Sounds Good, But . . .

It's making gold (for the book authors) out of ignorance.

—Dr. Jules Hirsch,
Rockefeller University Hospital

You may have heard of a new discovery, a "quick fix" that promises you'll lose weight easily and speedily. First, it's a low carbohydrate diet, but then a high carbohydrate diet promises to do the trick. Then there's the grapefruit diet, the cabbage soup diet, high protein diets, low protein diets, lowfat diets, high carbohydrate lowfat diets, very low calorie diets, liquid diets, diet drugs, and even think yourself thin programs. The list gets longer as trendy diets come and go while people waste their time and money chasing a dream of forever being thin. The search has been going on for many years.

How can you recognize a diet that's not reliable? Most make promises that sound too good to be true.

- The diet promises a quick weight loss of many pounds a week.
- The diet limits or avoids some foods.
- The diet allows you to eat as much as you want of some foods.

- The diet requires you to buy special foods.
- The diet promises that weight loss can be maintained without exercise or lifestyle changes.

High Protein, Low Carbohydrate Diets

High protein diets have been around since the 1970s and there's still no published research to support them. Supporters of these diets claim that calorie for calorie, low carbohydrate diets promote greater weight loss. On these diets, you can eat unlimited amounts of protein and fat—steak, bacon, eggs, chicken, fish, butter and oils. But some experts believe that a high protein, high fat diet is harmful. High protein intake overworks the kidneys and could damage them. High fat intake increases the risk for heart disease and some types of cancer.

Using a high protein, low carbohydrate diet for a month or two is harmless but, when it is continued over a longer period of time, the body may be thrown into an abnormal state known as ketosis. It is an unhealthy condition for everyone because it upsets the body's balance of water and electrolytes, disrupting blood pressure and kidney function. This is particularly dangerous if you have diabetes.

When you eat less calories and carbohydrates, the body uses stored glucose (sugar) for energy, releasing water as it is used. This water loss accounts for much of the weight loss. If you continue eating very little carbohydrates, the body starts to break down muscle. Therefore a high protein diet causes water and muscle loss but almost always, this weight loss is temporary. Bad breath, body odor, and constipation are other unpleasant side effects of a high protein diet. These diets work because they restrict variety and when there are fewer foods to eat, people get tired of eating the same foods over and over and so they eat less. A high protein intake strips calcium from your bones and can result in serious problems like osteoporosis (bone thinning). Some high protein diets are limited in other important vitamins and minerals. A very high intake of meat, fish and poultry can shortchange the amount of folic acid (a B vitamin) you are getting. This vitamin protects against birth defects and heart disease. In other words, eating high protein diets for a long time may cause serious health problems.

High Carbohydrate, Lowfat Diets

Fat is more calorie dense than carbohydrates. When you eat less fat, you eat fewer calories. This is the basis for high carbohydrate, lowfat diets. A teaspoon of fat has 45 calories, a teaspoon of carbohydrate has only 20. But if too many carbohydrate foods are eaten in place of fat, there may be no saving in calories. This often happens when people eat nonfat or lowfat foods that have lots of added sugar. Many experts believe Americans are gaining weight because of too many carbohydrates, especially sugar.

Celebrity Diet Books

These diets trade on the popularity of the "author," who is often a television or film personality. They usually have no professional credentials and the books are often based on unsubstantiated information. Basic assumptions of these diets often rest on "facts" that have no scientific support. Some of these diets claim you cannot mix different types of foods. Some give misleading information about digestive enzymes. Other diets tell you not to drink water with meals because it dilutes digestive juices and slows down digestion. All of this is incorrect.

Following most of these diets is not healthy, though you may see a short-term weight loss.

The Latest Diet Gimmick

Eat a grapefruit before every meal. Eat all the eggs you want. Feast one day, fast the next. Eat only raw foods. Have all the cabbage soup you want.

Over the last ten years the cabbage soup diet has appeared and reappeared in many forms. All are based on a seven-day cycle including cabbage soup made from cabbage, carrots, onions, celery, tomatoes, pepper, tomato juice, bouillon, and onion soup mix. The vegetables are healthy, but the onion soup mix and bouillon add a lot of salt. The Cabbage Soup Diet is not recommended by any health organizations. In fact, the American Heart Association has warned that the diet can be dangerous when people stay on it too long.

The diet is restrictive. On some days you can eat only certain foods like skim milk and bananas. Other days it's steak. Some days it's only cabbage soup. Eating the same foods, like cabbage soup on most days, becomes tiresome and less is eaten. The diet claims a weight loss of 10 to 15 pounds a week. This rapid weight loss will be short-lived because most of it is water that will be quickly replaced when you return to your regular eating habits. People who have tried the diet complained of feeling light-headed, weak, and suffering from upset stomach, gas and diarrhea. This diet also claims to clean impurities out of your system. Detoxification is a frequent claim in doubtful diets.

Carbohydrate Lover's Diets

Some trendy diet books blame foods that rapidly raise blood sugar for making people fat. Some carbohydrate foods have a high glycemic index, which triggers the release of insulin, thereby raising blood sugar. This causes more fat to be deposited in the body. This happens when you eat carbohydrate foods with a high glycemic index. But, because in everyday eating the carbohydrates we get are mixtures of high and low glycemic index foods, this does not happen on a regular basis.

Foods with a high glycemic index are sugar, honey, bagels, corn flakes, carrots, potatoes, white and whole wheat bread, and soft drinks. They are digested quickly, causing a rise in blood sugar. Foods with a low glycemic index break down more slowly and do not raise blood sugar quickly. Apples, beans, lentils, peaches, ice cream, yogurt, and peanuts are low glycemic index foods.

Using the glycemic index in weight loss has not been established because when foods are eaten together, the effect of the glycemic index is minimized. Experts believe that using the glycemic index may have value in controlling diabetes but it has little value in weight loss.

Food Combining

Other trendy diets claim that the wrong combinations of foods make you fat. There is no scientific truth to this. The basis of food-combining diets is that the enzymes in your body get confused when you eat certain combinations of food. Actually, the opposite is true. When your enzymes don't work correctly, *less* food is digested. The end result is that you would lose weight, not gain it.

There are many variations of food-combining diets. Some restrict certain foods completely. Others restrict foods to certain times of the day. For example, fruit may be eaten only before noon. Your stomach doesn't know what time it is. And it can handle any combination of foods at any time. In fact, almost all foods contain combinations of protein, carbohydrate and fat. Food combining and food restrictions are simply another way to eat less calories. There are healthier ways to do it.

Lose Weight While You Sleep

These well advertised products claim that when you take them right before going to bed, you lose weight overnight without changing your diet or adding exercise. Something that sounds this good couldn't possibly be true. You may have pleasant dreams, but you won't lose weight.

Diets in Cans or Bars

Walk into any supermarket, drugstore or convenience store and you're sure to find many different varieties of canned drinks and bars that are recommended to replace regular meals. The labels list the protein, fat, carbohydrate, vitamin and mineral content of these products, reassuring you that substituting one of these "meals" in a can or bar is the key to weight loss.

Many of the drinks taste pretty good and the bars look and taste very much like candy. That's because essentially they are shakes or candy bars with added vitamins and minerals! There's no harm in using these products once in a while. But eating them daily is a different story. They are not a substitute for real food. You'll feel cheated with the size of the "meal" and rarely feel satisfied. Drinking your lunch or eating a "candy bar" dinner once in a while won't hurt. It's just another way to get you to eat less calories. But they don't work in the long run. You won't learn how to face food and deal with it. Eating is something you'll be doing for a lifetime.

Take a Pill—Lose Weight

Ephedra (also known as ma huang), an herbal stimulant found in over 200 diet supplements, is used by millions of Americans for body-building and weight loss. Using it can be dangerous: ephedra has caused heart attacks, strokes, seizures, miscarriages, and deaths in healthy, young people. Other side effects include anxiety, insomnia, migraines, and high blood pressure.

Since the mid 1990s, there have been more than 54 deaths and 1,000 reports of complications linked to ephedra. According to Dr. Neal L. Benowitz, chief of clinical pharmacology at the University of California, "They're uncommon events, but they're serious. The substance is unreasonably hazardous as marketed." A recent study at the University of Arkansas concluded that labels on supplements containing ephedra are often misleading. Some brands contained potentially dangerous mixtures of ingredients and the amounts varied from one bottle to another.

The newest diet pills on the block contain chitosan, a dietary fiber made from the membranes and shells of shrimp and crabs. Chitosan can soak up 6 times its weight in fat, so absorption of some fat is prevented. The problem is that anything that stops the absorption of enough fat leads to gas, bloating and diarrhea when the bacteria in the intestines ferment the fat. Absorption of some vitamins is reduced as well. At this time, researchers are still arguing about the benefits. A much better way to lose weight is to eat less food.

A New Discovery . . . Based on What?

Dieting information is eagerly sought. When this information is presented by a well-known celebrity or seen in newspapers and magazines, it gains credibility at least for the moment, until newer information is announced.

But when sound scientific information is reported by the media it can be overwhelming. Often the public believes the researchers are changing their minds when they are simply reporting the results of new studies. Science is constantly evolving; new information becomes available all the time.

Get Skinny the Smart Way is based on sound, current scientific research. This research is described throughout the book. To lose weight and keep it off, you need to eat foods in commonsense amounts and you need to be physically active. We believe exercise is so important to control weight, it is a nonnegotiable part of the plan. Exercise not only burns calories but, it also uses up fat and promotes the building of muscles. The more muscle you have, the more calories you burn.

If you eat it and don't burn it, you sit on it.

Guidelines for a Good Diet

- It's based on current available research.

  The *Get Skinny* diet provides an extensive reference list beginning on page 351, listing the resources we used as the scientific foundation of the diet.
- It includes exercise.

  The *Get Skinny* diet believes activity is so important to weight loss that it is a nonnegotiable part of the diet.

- No foods are forbidden.

  It's not just the food you eat, but how much and how often you eat it. That is the reason you can't win the diet war. The *Get Skinny* diet will never ask you to fast, skip meals or give up any food. On *Get Skinny no foods are forbidden.*

- The diet does not use extreme measures.

  The *Get Skinny* diet will never ask you to have days when only liquids are allowed or a day when a specific food, like rice, is the only food eaten.

  You won't be told to use "special formulas" or pills to speed up your metabolism.

- The diet does not give you license to eat unlimited amounts of any food.

  Get Skinny's commonsense portions are the foundation of the thin eating habits you'll practice. Too much food, even when it is a healthy choice, is not good for you.

- The diet won't harm your health now or in the future.

  The *Get Skinny* diet, based on current, sound, scientific research, not only helps you lose weight but makes you healthier—you'll eat better and feel better.

- The diet has a plan for permanent weight maintenance.

  Get Skinny the Smart Way won't leave you stranded. Once you've reached your target weight, you'll move on to You're In Control—Maintaining Your Success in Chapter 11. *This is a diet you can live with for a lifetime.*

Chapter 4

Lose It Right

"Diet" is not a four-letter word that can't be said in public.

Mention the word "diet" and most of our clients shudder. They immediately think they'll have to endure an extended amount of time when they can't eat anything they enjoy. They believe they will be relegated to eating bland-tasting, tiny portions and unending bowls of "grass."

Diet by definition is "what a person usually eats." Granted, what you usually eat may be what got you where you are right now: weighing too much. But "diet" is not the culprit. It's just a word. We could put you on a diet to actually *gain weight* or we could put you on a diet to manage diabetes or high blood pressure.

We want you to try the *Get Skinny* diet, "what a healthy person usually eats," to help you achieve the weight loss you've always dreamed of and to help you become a healthier, fitter person. Why is *Get Skinny* different?

First of all, it's fun. We believe that eating should be fun— a regularly recurring pleasure you look forward to. Second, it works because we don't stop you from eating any foods. On the contrary, *no foods are forbidden.* We help you to implement thin habits and understand commonsense portions so that you can enjoy any food any time. Third, we introduce you to some remarkably simple fat and calorie burners that work. And, fourth, we get you moving. Active people burn calories more efficiently and therefore can eat more than inactive people.

What Research Told Us

Sometimes research tells us exactly what we think it will; other times we are in for big surprises. The biggest surprise of the last decade was that as the American public embraced the idea of eating less fat, they got fatter. Sounds like a contradiction, but it wasn't. Today, 97 million men, women and children in America are too heavy!

If fat wasn't making people fat, what was? The answers were portion sizes that grew out of control and an epidemic of inactivity. The original two-ounce hamburger, introduced in the 1950s by the first hamburger chain, has grown to a "whopping" double patty with cheese, averaging 600 calories. If you add to that a colossal-size order of fries—another 500 calories—and unlimited drink refills, followed by a few hours of "surfing" the Net, it's no wonder Americans are "spreading out" in all directions. Nearly two-thirds of Americans get no regular exercise and 25% never exercise.

This lack of activity and increase in portion sizes happened so quietly that the damage was done before experts realized what was happening. USDA statistics show that we are eating 148 more calories each day, on average, than we did 20 years ago. That may not sound like much, but it works out to an extra 15 pounds a year.

Obesity and inactivity are costing American taxpayers billions every year. Carrying around extra pounds is taking lives, an estimated 300,000 premature deaths a year. And weighing too much is making us sick, contributing to cases of heart disease, diabetes, cancer and possibly even infertility.

Everyone is scrambling to fix the problem or, at the very least, stop it from getting worse. The federal government, public health organizations, professional associations and education policy makers have all banded together to wage an all-out assault on America's quickly spreading epidemic. But, policy makers, as well-meaning as they might be, move slowly. Like most people we talk to every day, you are not willing to wait a decade for the government to get effective programs in place. You want to lose weight now!

A Closer Look at You

We've never believed in the "one-size-fits-all" approach to weight control. Each of you, and the lives you lead, is unique. For a weight loss plan to work it has to fit you. One of the best things about *Get Skinny* is that it can be tailored for you like a custom-made suit.

You'll begin, in Chapter 7, by taking a closer look at you. You'll examine your diet history, weight history, health risks, activity level, and how you currently eat. Next you'll set goals: a target weight, a target calorie zone and a weekly activity goal designed just for you.

Our Contribution

We'll be your ally. Every time you have a question, come up against a problem you don't know how to handle, or need to modify your eating plan or activity goals, we'll help you do it.

Begin Where You Wish

As former college teachers we always hoped our students would read every book we assigned from cover to cover. We hope you'll read every chapter of *Get Skinny the Smart Way* because we believe each one is loaded with valuable information that will make you smarter and more capable of winning the weight war once and for all. But it isn't necessary to wait to start losing weight until you've read the entire book. We appreciate how anxious you are to get started.

Begin by reading Chapter 7, A Closer Look at You. Go on to Chapters 5 and 6, where you'll find out about *Get Skinny's* fabulous dieting aids—pectin, calcium and water—and the 3 important secrets to your success—thin habits, the power of portion and the enjoyment of exercise. In Chapter 8, you'll discover how to face food fearlessly. Now you are ready to begin losing weight with the help of the **Smart Start** phase of the *Get Skinny* diet in Chapter 9. At this point, you can take some time and read Chapters 1, 2 and 3 to learn more about the background and development of the *Get Skinny* diet. Chapter 10, Moving Along, is the second phase of the diet. By the time you get to Chapter 11, You're In Control, you'll have reached your target weight and, at this point, we'll arm you with more information to ensure your continued success. Chapter 12, Take a Bow!, is graduation, where you assess how far you've come. When you get there, you'll hear us clapping loudly to celebrate your success.

Smart Start

We developed the **Smart Start** phase of the *Get Skinny* diet to assure you a quick, substantial weight loss. You want results and you'll get them during the 28 days of **Smart Start**.

We know how difficult it is to change many behaviors at once, so during **Smart Start** we'll be working as a team. We'll plan all the meals while you concentrate on practicing *thin habits* and becoming more active. Slowly, we'll put you in charge.

With 3 meals and 3 snacks a day, some of our clients feel that **Smart Start** contains too much food. They're wrong. Research has shown that eating commonsense portions at regular intervals throughout the day, is key to losing weight and maintaining the loss. Trust us, this works.

In **Smart Start**, you'll also be using *Get Skinny's* powerful dieting aids—pectin, calcium and water. Pectin is a fiber made from apples and grapefruit. It can be bought at the supermarket in powdered form. Added to food it makes you feel fuller for a longer period of time. *Pectin power!* Food consumption surveys continuously demonstrate that people with the lowest calcium intakes weigh the most. Adequate calcium is essential for good health and too few of us get enough. It also explains why so many of us are overweight. The *Get Skinny* diet is planned so that you'll never fall short of calcium again. *Calcium counts!* Water, with no calories, burns calories. How? When you have too little water your body slows down and uses up calories less quickly. When you drink enough water you burn calories more efficiently. *Water works!*

Moving Along

Moving Along is the second phase of *Get Skinny*. You'll stay with this phase until you've reached your target weight. Many of our clients use this phase as their model for lifelong eating. Perhaps you will, too. Based on your own individualized target calorie zone, in **Moving Along,** you'll be setting up an eating plan that is suited to your lifestyle, likes and dislikes.

By now, you'll have grown accustomed to incorporating *Get Skinny*'s powerful dieting aids into your day. You'll be so good at using *thin habits* that, on most days, you'll not have to think about them consciously. You'll be able to estimate commonsense portion sizes like a pro, and you'll be healthier and more active than you've ever been before. You'll definitely be *moving along* toward your target weight.

You're in Charge

One of the most important goals of the *Get Skinny* diet is to put you in charge. Once you've reached your target weight and you're physically fit, you'll want to stay that way. Old friends are loyal; they don't abandon you. At this point the *Get Skinny* diet will be a loyal, old friend continuing to offer you strategies to maintain your weight loss and stay active for the rest of your life.

Data collected by the National Weight Control Registry from real people, just like you, who have lost weight and kept it off for years, shows that these weight loss success stories sound just like yours. The successful losers followed a sensible eating plan without gimmicks. So will you. They changed their eating and exercise habits. So will you. They kept their weight off for years by incorporating the changes they made into their everyday life. So will you. There is no question, you'll be in charge!

Exercise

Successful weight loss and its long term maintenance can't be accomplished without exercise. Don't throw the book down and run screeching from the room when you read this. As with everything in this diet, your exercise program will be tailored to you. Our only goal is to get you to *move*.

You'll decide on the actual activity. It can be real life fitness—things you do every day that burn calories. It can be walking. Or, it can be a structured exercise class or program. You choose, you move, you lose!

In Chapter 6, Appendix 1 and Appendix 2, we've provided all the information you'll need to get going—how to start exercising, how to track the calories you burn, and a basic stretching and strength-training program. Whether you are a full-time couch potato or you already lead an active life, this information will refocus your activity into a major calorie-burning force that will help you lose weight faster and keep it off. Not only will you be slimmer and fitter, you'll be healthier. In addition to helping you lose weight, exercise is a powerful weapon against aging and the risk for serious illness.

And There's More . . .

Over the years—by working as professionals, teaching, and answering people's questions—we've collected a tremendous amount of information. As a way to share some of that "extra" information with you, you will come across **Smart Stuff** boxes scattered throughout the book. "Stuff" that might make you laugh, an odd fact that's interesting, some technical information, a research finding, or a practical tip to add to your bag of tricks. Smart Stuff we wanted you to know.

You'll also find special features in each chapter—rating quizzes, charts, lists, tables, worksheets—all designed to put the information you need at your fingertips. In Chapter 9 you'll find a hunger and a satisfaction scale. They will help you get in touch with your body's food signals. In Chapter 10 we've shared questions people have asked us about losing weight. The answers will help you over trouble spots.

We've also included recipes throughout the book. All of them fit into your diet, taste good, and are quick and easy to prepare. The calories in one serving are listed with each recipe and are also listed in Appendix 3, which gives the serving size and calories of over 600 foods.

Starting *Your Personalized Weight Attack Plan*

Get Skinny the Smart Way

1. Take **A Closer Look at You** in Chapter 7 (page 100). It's important to know where you're coming from before you know where you're going. You'll establish jumping-off points for your individualized eating and exercise program.

2. Find out more about:

   Get Skinny's **Fabulous Dieting Aids** in Chapter 5 (page 34)
   Pectin Power (page 35)
   Calcium Counts (page 40)
   Water Works (page 44)

   Get Skinny's Secrets to Success in Chapter 6 (page 48)
   Thin Habits (page 49)
   The Power of Portions (page 61)
   Exercise (page 85)

3. Use Chapter 9 (page 171) **Smart Start** to begin losing and moving today!

Chapter 5

Let Nature Help You Do It—Powerful Dieting Aids

It's the next best thing to magic . . . dieting aids that work.

Your Personalized Weight Attack Plan will introduce you to three surprising, powerful dieting allies that will help you reach your target weight. By incorporating these hunger chasers and calorie burners into your everyday eating plans, you'll find it easy to drop pounds while never feeling hungry or deprived and you'll stay healthy.

Pectin Power—hunger chaser

Calcium Counts—calorie burner

Water Works—calorie burner

Dieting Gone Wrong

When you see "before" and "after" pictures of someone who lost pounds simply by drinking liquid meals, taking an appetite suppressant or even wearing a special bracelet, it's very tempting. You want to rush out to get a dieting aid that is guaranteed to drop those extra pounds. It sounds good but, before you take the plunge, be aware that you may lose only time and money. And you could be harming your health.

In November 2000, the Food and Drug Administration (FDA) banned the sale of diet pills, cough medicines and cold remedies that contain phenylpropanolamine (PPA). Although this nonprescription drug has been in use for over fifty years, recent evidence from many reports found that PPA increases the risk of stroke (bleeding in the brain) causing disability and death. The FDA has estimated that PPA caused 200 to 500 strokes in people under 50. In 44 stroke cases among PPA users tracked by the FDA in the past 30 years, most were women with an average age of 35 using PPA-containing dieting aids. The actual number of strokes is probably more than 1,000, because few were actually reported. Other serious reactions to PPA are convulsions, kidney failure, heart damage, severe headache and high blood pressure. What's most important is the lack of evidence that using dieting aids containing PPA helped people lose weight and keep it off. But there is evidence of dangerous side effects.

There are safer ways to slim down and stay healthy. *Get Skinny*'s powerful dieting allies—pectin, calcium, water—will help you to lose weight without harm.

PECTIN POWER

Get Skinny's Pectin Goal:

One pectin-containing food or drink a day
as a hunger chaser.

Our clients love pectin. It's a powerful hunger chaser when you are trying to lose weight. Pectin isn't anything mysterious. You've been eating it all your life without realizing it. Every time you eat an apple, apricot, peach, pear, plum, prune, raisins, strawberries, raspberries, raw carrot, raw onion, sweet potato or beans, you get some pectin. Orange, lemon and grapefruit peels also contain pectin as does jelly and most reduced calorie yogurts.

Pectin is a carbohydrate and a source of dietary fiber that has no calories. It passes through the body without being absorbed, helping to reduce cholesterol, blood sugar levels, and the risk of colon cancer. It's an ingredient used to thicken foods and is found in medicines to treat diarrhea. Pectin is good for you.

Pectin slows down the emptying of your stomach, making you feel fuller longer. Simply adding pectin to foods like yogurt, juice, applesauce, and cooked cereal does the trick. Because you feel fuller for a longer period of time you eat less.

SMART STUFF

A study done at Brooke Army Medical Center in Texas compared subjects given orange juice with added pectin to other subjects given just plain orange juice. They found that, regardless of the amount of pectin added to the juice, those who had the pectin-containing drink felt fuller for up to four hours after drinking it. As little as 1 teaspoon of pectin makes you feel fuller.

Where to Find Pectin

Pectin is available at the supermarket in two forms—powdered and liquid. Sure-Jel, a powdered pectin and Certo, a liquid, are two nationally distributed brands. Regional brands of pectin are also available. Look in the aisle where the pudding mixes and baking supplies are shelved or where canning supplies are found. Pectin is usually made from apples and grapefruit. Pure apple and grapefruit pectin can be found in health food stores in tablets or as a powder.

How to Use Pectin

Pectin is powerful at relieving hunger when added to foods. Make a pectin cocktail by stirring 1 teaspoon of pectin into a glass of lemonade, orange juice, tomato juice or seltzer. Pectin can be stirred into any drink you enjoy—even diet soda—without adding taste. Add the pectin right before you drink it. If you prefer the consistency of a smoothie, let your drink stand for a few minutes to thicken. But pectin does not have to thicken food to work as a hunger chaser.

Pectin is a source of fiber so it's important to slowly add it to your diet. It's best not to use too much too soon. During the first two weeks you are on the *Get Skinny* diet, you'll be gradually increasing the amount of pectin you add to food from 1 teaspoon to 3 teaspoons (1 tablespoon) a day. We recommend a maximum limit of 1 tablespoon a day mixed into a drink or stirred into yogurt.

Pectin can be added to many foods. Stir it into yogurt or applesauce—it makes the yogurt more creamy and custardy and the applesauce thicker and smoother. Other fruit sauces are good as well. Pectin can also be added to soup, mashed potatoes, or cooked cereal, like oatmeal or Cream of Wheat. Adding pectin slows down the emptying of your stomach, dulls your appetite and increases your feeling of fullness. You can keep single serving fruit sauces and powdered pectin in your desk drawer. Use it to take the edge off your appetite before a business lunch or dinner on the town.

The Scoop on Other Fibers

Pectin is just one member of the fiber family. Fiber is an important part of *Your Personalized Weight Attack Plan*. Experts recommend you eat 25 to 35 grams of fiber every day, but Americans average only 10 to 15. That's less than half the recommended amount. The *Get Skinny* diet encourages you to eat food high in fiber to help fill you up without filling you out.

Fiber has other benefits as well. It protects your heart, prevents constipation, helps control diabetes, and lowers cholesterol. Some studies show that vegetables, citrus fruits, and high fiber grains reduce the risk for colon cancer. It's obvious that, in general, Americans need to eat more fiber.

SMART STUFF

A study done at the Institute of Physiology, University of Lausanne, Switzerland found that eating a high fiber meal reduced feelings of hunger more so than a low fiber meal. The researchers believe that a high fiber intake would help people have better control of the amount of food they eat.

Fiber is found in plants: leaves (spinach), stems (asparagus), flowers (cauliflower), roots (carrots) and seeds (peas). The amount of fiber goes up as the plant grows. Fruits and vegetables, eaten with their peel, and whole grain breads and cereals provide even more fiber. Whole grains include whole wheat flour and bread, brown rice, popcorn and oatmeal. High fiber foods are usually very low in fat. They take longer to chew. They fill up your stomach without adding calories. Fiber passes through the body and is not digested.

It's Easy to Eat More Fiber

- Eat whole wheat bread and whole grain cereals.
- Top any cereal with 1 or 2 tablespoons of bran or wheat germ.
- Eat the skin on fruits and vegetables.
- Eat meatless meals—eating fruits, grains and vegetables instead.
- Eat less meat—it has no fiber.
- Eat beans a couple of times a week.
- Add beans and peas to soups, salads, and casseroles.
- Add pectin to yogurt, juice, cooked cereal or any food.

SMART STUFF

"The concentration of dietary fiber in most foods is low. The best way to increase intake . . . is to consume *more servings* of fiber-containing foods."

—Judith A. Marlett, Ph.D., R.D.
University of Wisconsin–Madison

To Get the Most Fiber

Eat This	Instead of This
Whole wheat bread	White bread
	Wheat bread
	Rye bread
Baked potato with skin	Mashed potatoes
	French fries
Brown rice	White rice
Beans	Rice
Lentils	
Peas	
Oatmeal	Cream of Wheat
Wheatena	Cream of Rice
Corn	Grits
	Polenta
All vegetables	Vegetable juice
All fruits	Fruit juice
Graham crackers	Cookies
Popcorn	Chips
Whole grain crackers	Plain crackers
Raisin bran	Frosted Flakes
Shredded Wheat	Corn Flakes
Grape-nuts	Puffed Rice
Cheerios	Puffed Wheat
Kashi	Rice Krispies
Cracklin' Oat Bran	
Whole wheat pasta	Regular pasta
Buckwheat (soba) noodles	Egg noodles

Smart Stuff

Start with soup is a thin habit. Adding 1 to 3 teaspoons of pectin will double the benefit.

CALCIUM COUNTS

Get Skinny's **Calcium Goal:**

Two servings of lowfat calcium-rich foods plus a
600 milligram (mg) calcium supplement daily.

Calcium is a powerful ally in helping you lose weight. Recent research shows that the risk for obesity is highest in people with the lowest calcium intake. Researchers at the University of Tennessee did an analysis of NHANES III (the third National Health and Nutrition Examination Survey) and found that people with the lowest intake of calcium were 6 times more likely to be obese. And the risk of being significantly overweight went down as calcium intake went up.

Animal studies done in the same laboratory showed that low amounts of calcium increase body fat. When calcium levels are low, hormones that tell the body to hold on to and store extra fat increase. The researchers wondered if extra calcium, added to a low calorie diet, would help very fat mice lose weight. It did. These studies are currently being repeated with people to see if they have the same result.

SMART STUFF

Adequate vitamin D is needed for absorption of calcium. Studies show that obese people have low levels of vitamin D in their blood. Most of this vitamin is obtained from sunlight and overweight people tend to avoid sun exposure. Vitamin D is also available from some fortified foods, like milk and cereals, and from vitamin supplements.

On the *Get Skinny* diet we are recommending adequate calcium because it has many benefits in addition to weight loss. It seems that weight gain can be added to a long list of serious health problems associated with low calcium intakes—osteoporosis (bone thinning), high blood pressure, PMS (premenstrual syndrome), colon cancer and kidney stones. That's why we encourage our clients to eat two servings of lowfat calcium-rich foods and take a calcium supplement of 600 milligrams every day. This will help you lose weight, slow down bone loss and protect you from serious health risks.

SMART STUFF

Many fad diets shortchange dieters when it comes to calcium, cutting calcium-rich foods to cut calories. This could lead to increased bone thinning (osteoporosis), especially in women.

Best Sources of Calcium

Milk, yogurt and cheese are loaded with calcium. You'll find that many other foods like cottage cheese, orange juice, and cereal have extra calcium added. Whenever you can, choose reduced fat or nonfat versions of milk, yogurt and cheese. These cut calories while giving you the calcium you need.

Leafy, green vegetables like spinach, broccoli, collards, and turnip greens are rich in calcium. Other good sources are beans, and canned sardines or salmon, when they are eaten with their soft bones. Calcium-containing mineral water is another good source. Enjoy fun foods: cappuccino, latte, shakes, and smoothies made with lowfat milk, and frozen lowfat yogurt are also high in calcium.

Getting Enough Calcium

On *Your Personalized Weight Attack Plan,* you get enough calcium to help you lose weight and protect your health. You get the calcium you need in two ways—from food and from supplements. The *Get Skinny* diet recommends two servings a day of lowfat, calcium-rich foods plus a 600 milligram (mg) calcium supplement.

Getting Two Servings of Calcium-Rich Food Each Day

- Add nonfat milk to your cereal.
- Eat lowfat or nonfat yogurt often.
- Eat lowfat or nonfat frozen yogurt.
- Eat reduced fat cheese.
- Eat lowfat or nonfat calcium-fortified cottage cheese.
- Choose calcium-fortified juice.
- Choose calcium-fortified foods.
- Eat green, leafy vegetables often.
- Eat canned salmon or sardines.

Calcium in Food

Food	Amount	Milligrams Calcium
Nonfat milk	1 cup	300
Calcium-fortified orange juice	1 cup	300
Yogurt	1 snack-size	100–200
Yogurt	1 container	200–400
Cheese	1 ounce	100–150
Vanilla ice cream	½ cup	100–150
Vanilla frozen yogurt	½ cup	100–400
Nonfat ricotta cheese	½ cup	200–300
Nonfat cottage cheese	½ cup	100–200

You'll notice that many foods you usually eat are now calcium-fortified. You can use these as 1 or 2 of your calcium-rich servings each day. You'll get the rest of the calcium you need from a supplement.

Many of our clients stop taking their calcium supplement after they reach their target weight. They eat more calcium-rich foods instead. You'll decide this for yourself later on. In the meantime, we'll help you pick a calcium supplement.

Many brands and dosages of calcium are available. The most common supplement is calcium carbonate, usually made from oyster shells. It is well absorbed, inexpensive, and the pills are small enough to be swallowed easily. Calcium citrate malate and calcium gluconate are other calcium supplements you can try.

They are bulkier. This means that you'll have to take more pills or larger pills to get enough calcium. Another option—calcium chews—are becoming widely available.

SMART STUFF

It's a good idea to spread out your calcium-rich foods and supplements throughout the day. This helps increase their absorption. Some experts suggest taking calcium at bedtime because it is absorbed while you sleep.

Too much of a good thing is not always better. Getting over 2,500 milligrams of calcium a day, from foods and supplements, may be more than is good for you. High calcium intakes can also interfere with the absorption of other minerals such as iron and zinc. Taking too much calcium can cause constipation and, sometimes, kidney stones.

Choosing and Using a Calcium Supplement

- Select a supplement that provides 600 milligrams of calcium.
- We recommend a calcium supplement that contains vitamin D.
- Choose a supplement that states "essentially lead free" on the label.
- For better absorption, take your calcium supplement with a meal.
- Do not take a calcium supplement along with other minerals such as iron, zinc and manganese. Calcium interferes with their absorption.

SMART STUFF—Get the lead out

Some calcium supplements may contain an unsafe amount of lead. There are brands of calcium supplements labeled "essentially lead-free." ConsumerLab.com is an independent testing lab that evaluates calcium supplements and lists those that are safe.

WATER WORKS
Get Skinny's Water Goal:
A total of 8 to 10 glasses of water and other liquids each day

Water is a powerful calorie burner. It helps you lose weight. Researchers at the University of Utah in Salt Lake City found that when you have too little water in the body, your metabolism slows down and you burn fewer calories. Exercising, running errands and staying out in the sunshine is enough to dehydrate your body. Drinking plenty of water and other liquids to keep your body hydrated helps burn more calories.

Researchers at Penn State found that drinking water also aids in controlling hunger. Eating fruits and vegetables that contain a lot of water, such as watermelon or celery, is another way to reduce hunger and starting a meal with water or soup cuts down on the number of calories you consume.

Are You Really Hungry or Just Thirsty?

Sometimes, when you think you're hungry, your body may actually be signaling for water, not food. The next time you feel hungry, try a large glass of water and see if you feel satisfied. You may be surprised to find that you were just thirsty.

SMART STUFF

Seventy-three percent of your body is water. That equals 10 gallons. People can survive for weeks without food, but only a few days without fluids. You lose about 1 gallon of water a day and need to take in that much to replace it. Over your lifetime, you'll drink about 100,000 gallons of water!

How Much Water Is Enough?

Your Personalized Weight Attack Plan recommends that you drink 8 to 10 glasses of water and other liquids every day. That sounds like a lot, but we're recommending an 8 ounce glass. Most water glasses hold 10 to 12 ounces. A recent survey conducted by Rockefeller University in New York City and the International Bottled Water Association found that only 34% of Americans drink the recommended 8 glasses of water a day. Nearly 10% say they drink no water at all. Your body loses water continuously during the day and night. This needs to be replaced, and you can't wait until you're thirsty to decide that you need water—at this point your body is already dehydrated.

SMART STUFF
75% of Americans are chronically dehydrated.

Water, juices, seltzer, mineral water, milk and caffeine-free coffee, tea, and soda all contribute to your fluid total. Choose drinks that are not heavily sweetened because they add too many calories.

Alcohol, soda, beer and regular coffee and tea dehydrate you and cause you to lose water. Many experts recommend one glass of water for every glass of soda or cup of coffee you drink. This may be going too far because these drinks don't cause you to lose all of the water you drink. We'd take a more moderate approach. Don't count alcohol as a source of water, but you can count half of the coffee, tea and soda you drink as water. Therefore, one cup of coffee or one glass of soda each equals a half cup of water.

SMART STUFF
If you don't urinate at least every four hours when you are awake, you probably need to be drinking more.

Making Water Work to Help You Lose Pounds

- Drinking water along with high fiber foods helps the fiber expand in your stomach. This will make you feel fuller longer without adding calories. Have popcorn and seltzer as a TV snack.

- Eating foods with a high water content will reduce the amount of calories you eat. Snack on watermelon. Have sherbet for dessert.
- When you feel hungry, have a large glass of water first. Set the kitchen timer for 10 to 15 minutes and get busy doing something you enjoy. If you're still hungry when the timer goes off, try another glass of water before you eat.
- When your body is well hydrated, it speeds up your metabolism so you burn more calories and lose more weight.
- If you like sweet drinks, choose diet soda, diet lemonade or diet fruit drinks.
- Enjoy a cup or two of green tea every day.
- Make sure you drink at least 8 glasses of water or other beverages each day.

Green Tea, a Fat Burner

There are many types of tea to choose from, but green tea has special benefits when you are trying to lose weight. Tea is more than just a refreshing drink—it's a fat burner. It is practically calorie-free, has a pleasant, mild taste, and the antioxidants in tea help prevent cancer and heart disease. Studies using an extract of green tea showed that it burned fat and calories and subjects in the study lost weight. Researchers at the University of Geneva in Switzerland found that antioxidants in green tea increase metabolism and fat burning so that more calories are used. Subjects who were given green tea used up more calories than those who took a placebo.

Green tea can be bought loose or in teabags. Some brands offer flavored green tea as well. The best way to brew green tea is simple: pour boiling water into an empty tea cup; let the water stand a minute to cool; add the green tea and steep for one minute. Making time for a healthy tea break during your busy day will boost your metabolism and burn fat quicker.

Get Skinny *Goals for Your Personalized Weight Attack Plan*

Pectin—hunger chaser

Add 1 to 3 teaspoons of pectin to food each day as a hunger chaser.

Calcium—calorie burner

2 servings of calcium-rich foods—and— a 600 milligram calcium supplement each day.

Water—calorie burner

8 to 10 glasses of water and other liquids each day.

Chapter 6

Secrets to Your Success

We have to de-normalize high-calorie, low-fiber diets and inactivity.

—Dileep Bal, M.P.H., M.D.,
Cancer Control Branch,
California Department of Health Services

Everybody has a skinny friend who they love to hate. It's that person who never seems to give a second thought to food. The person whose dress size hasn't changed in years. What is their secret?

People who are slim do have secrets to share. In this chapter we are going to look at some of these secrets we've learned by observing the habits of slim people. How much they eat. When they eat. What they eat. How much they move. These secrets will become yours and you will put them into action to reach your target weight.

There is a lot of information to "digest" in this chapter (pardon the pun). 1. Understanding **thin habits** and integrating them into your day-to-day eating routine. 2. Estimating **portion sizes** accurately so you don't overeat. 3. Incorporating **activity** into every day. Read the chapter through once but don't expect to remember everything. Come back to it again and again to reinforce the ideas, attitudes and behaviors recommended. Before you know it you will have incorporated so many weight loss "secrets" into your daily life that soon you'll be one of those skinny people you've envied for so long.

THIN HABITS

Habit—a thing done so often it becomes easy.

—Webster's Dictionary

Thin habits are eating behaviors that slim people use, instinctively, to keep their weight in check. Thin habits will help put your appetite and eating style into slow motion so that you'll overeat less and get more satisfaction from food. Thin eating habits can be grouped into three main categories—when to eat, how to eat, what to eat.

When to Eat

Eat when you're hungry.

Sounds obvious, right? But most of our overweight clients truly cannot define the sensation of "hunger." All they know is when it's lunchtime or, they eat to satisfy something other than hunger. Food can substitute for companionship. Sometimes they eat out of boredom, frustration or to relieve stress.

Slim people, on the other hand, actually feel hungry. It's been long enough since they've eaten that their body is signaling them to refuel with more food. Some describe it as a gnawing in their stomach or a feeling of emptiness; sometimes the stomach rumbles or growls.

If you've lost touch with your sense of hunger, it is a feeling we want you to regain. In Smart Start, we'll be planning your meals and snacks. You'll practice regular refueling (eating) at specific times and we'll get you to ignore those external cues that tell you to eat for other reasons. From now on, every time you want to eat, ask yourself this simple question, "Am I hungry?." If the answer is, "I want a break from my desk"; "That TV commercial was very enticing"; "My husband and I just had a disagreement"; "The kids are driving me nuts!"; or "The bagel shop smells delicious," you probably aren't truly hungry but are being driven to eat by an external cue. This exercise is not always guaranteed to stop you from eating but it will slow you down and make you think about why you are eating. And that is the whole idea behind thin habits: to get you to think about food differently.

Eat regular meals plus a snack or two.

Eating frequently does not equal overeating. On the contrary, small frequent meals lead to more satisfaction than a few large ones. Plan a snack break rather than spontaneously grabbing something between meals. Consider snacks an extension of the last meal or a warm-up for the next. Instead of dessert after dinner, plan a snack in the evening. Fresh fruit midmorning could complement a small breakfast. A small salad or a mug of soup, midafternoon, could be a pre-dinner satisfier.

Eat breakfast.

Your body needs fuel in the morning to *break* the long night's *fast* without food. Eating breakfast puts your body in gear so you burn calories faster than if you don't eat until lunch. Studies have proven that breakfast eaters are leaner, have lower blood pressure and get a wider variety of nutrients daily than breakfast skippers. Research on cognition and dexterity give higher marks to those who eat an A.M. meal. But a 1999 survey showed that more than 60% of us don't eat breakfast. If a morning meal is not your cup of tea, try being inventive—a sandwich, cottage cheese and fruit, a container of yogurt, even pizza is okay. What you eat is not important; it's more important that you eat. Having breakfast is a thin habit.

Skip the midnight feeding.

Your body is more likely to store calories eaten late at night because you are less likely to use up this extra energy with activity. Sometimes a bedtime snack is a holdover from childhood. If you depend on this to feel sleepy, try switching to a cup of herbal tea. Late night refrigerator raids are often triggered by emotions. Examine your motives; are you really hungry?

How to Eat

Eat slowly.

It takes time for your stomach to signal your brain that you are full. Recently, a team of scientists from the University of Florida and the University of Texas determined that it takes at least 10 minutes for a feeling of fullness to be processed by the brain. It may take even longer for people who are significantly overweight. The researchers theorized that extra pounds may impair or damage this message system.

You can use a number of thin habits to slow down your appetite while you wait for the "full" sign. Note the time you started eating and stretch the meal out to last at least 10 minutes. Sip water or another no-calorie beverage between bites. Put your fork down between bites. Swallow each mouthful completely before you take another bite. Talk to your meal companion—you won't hold a conversation with food in your mouth.

Want dessert? Wait 10 minutes before you order. You might find that you're already full and no longer want, or need, the chocolate cake you were about to order.

Leave serving dishes on the counter or stove.

Don't put serving dishes on the table. Getting up to take seconds requires more time and effort than just reaching for a spoon. This simple thin habit creates a pause in the meal that might be just long enough to help you think about whether you are still hungry or not. You're probably not!

Eat from plates, not packages.

Nibbling from a package of chips or spooning ice cream directly from the carton is a recipe for overeating. Use a plate, serve out a portion and put the package away.

Eat at the table.

Simply telling our clients not to eat while doing another activity can cut hundreds of calories a day! Think about it—when was the last time you saw a new car without a cup holder? There is a candy store next to most bus and subway stops. Malls have food courts and ice cream shops. Bookstores serve coffee and cake. It's far too easy to eat as you move through your day. Sitting and eating at a table—no more eating in the car, munching in the lounge chair in front of the TV, or snacking in bed—is one of the simplest thin habits you can use to stop overeating.

SMART STUFF

Marketers encourage you to eat on-the-go by producing food items they refer to as "hyperconvenience," "portable comfort food," or "dashboard dining." Any food that can be shaped or packaged to fit into a car cup holder or eaten utensil-less straight from the package has a marketing advantage. Many of those currently available are high in sodium, fat and sugar and low in fruits and vegetables.

Quit the clean plate club.

Many of us were encouraged to eat every bit of food on our plates, even if we were full. We were told by well-meaning parents, "People are starving!." Those same people are still starving while you pack on extra pounds by cleaning your plate. You aren't alone—over 50% of adults clean their plates, even when they're full. When you feel satisfied, you've eaten enough. Slim people do this without thinking. Listen to your body. Let it tell you when to stop regardless of how much is left on your plate. To get this **thin habit** going, make a conscious effort to leave a few bites behind at first. As time goes on, you'll get better at "hearing" your body's signals and it will be easier to stop once you've had enough.

Resist the "Now I've blown it!" syndrome.

No one is perfect. So you ate the whole piece of cheesecake, so what! One large meal, one dessert, one bag of chips did not make you overweight. It was one large meal after another, one too many desserts, and far too many bags of chips. All too often, when you are trying to lose weight, you either stick to your diet strictly or you blow it by overindulging. This all-or-nothing approach rarely works because you end up spending more time cheating and feeling guilty than trying to establish new thin habits. Anyone who is trying to make a significant lifestyle change will backslide every now and then. Don't waste time beating yourself up, just re-institute thin habits and get going in the right direction again.

Keep food out of sight, out of reach.

Candy dishes, cookie jars, and open bags of chips on the counter all spell temptation. Put all food out of sight, in covered containers, so you cannot snatch a snack spontaneously. Purge the house of your hidden reserves—peanuts in the den, cookies in the nightstand, candy in the desk drawer—and keep all food in the kitchen.

SMART STUFF

A good night's sleep can control your appetite. Researchers at Colorado State University at Fort Collins found that peoples' appetites soared when they were sleep-deprived. Getting enough sleep is a thin habit.

What to Eat

Start with soup.

Studies have shown that soup can curb your appetite for the food that follows. Researchers at Pennsylvania State University showed that women who began lunch with soup ate fewer calories at that meal. Soup is warm and fragrant. It takes time to eat a bowlful and you feel you have been offered a substantial portion of food. All this adds up to satisfaction. Choose clear broths, noodle, vegetable or bean soups rather than bisques, creamed or cheese-topped options to keep the satisfaction high and the calories low.

SMART STUFF

Consider a warm mug of broth as a midafternoon or evening TV snack. Even if you add a few crackers, it's still a smart choice.

More fruits and vegetables, less juice.

A study at the Energy Metabolism Laboratory at Tufts University showed that people who ate a wide variety of fruits and vegetables were leaner. Sounds obvious, but this was the first time that researchers actually showed an association between dietary variety and body fat. Eating a number of fruits and vegetables on a daily basis is a thin habit. Yet just five vegetables—fresh potatoes, frozen potatoes, onions, iceberg lettuce and canned tomatoes—make up half of all the vegetables we regularly eat. Though juices are healthy choices, they are more calorie dense and don't offer the chewing satisfaction of the whole fruit or vegetable. Until you reach your target weight it is wiser to "chew" than "drink" your fruit and vegetable choices.

Curb calories in a glass.

According to researchers at Purdue University, liquid calories don't register the same feeling of fullness as solid food. Drinking one can of soda or juice a day, which typically contains about 120 calories, adds up to 12 extra pounds in a year. Coffee laced with cream, fruit smoothies, milkshakes, beer, mixed drinks, sweetened ice tea and even good-for-you fruit juice can add more calories than you realize. Until you reach your target weight stick to no-calorie drinks like water, mineral water, seltzer, diet soda, and unsweetened tea.

SMART STUFF

Freeze any fruit juice you enjoy in ice cube trays and use the fruit cubes to chill seltzer, mineral water, or diet ginger ale— a flavor and nutrient boost with very few calories.

Fat free doesn't equal calorie free.

Cookies, candies, chips, ice cream, dips, and salad dressings are just a few of the thousands of "fat free" goodies that line the supermarket shelf. Many of these new products are loaded with sugar and can pack quite a calorie wallop. It's okay to eat these, just as long as you keep portion sizes moderate. A box of "fat free" cookies is not a serving!

Fill up on fiber.

Foods high in fiber—fruits, vegetables, whole grain cereals and bread, brown rice, whole wheat pasta, beans—offer less calories coupled with the satisfaction of chewing. As you know from Chapter 5, fiber is a great dieting aid. Regularly choosing high fiber foods is a thin habit.

Buy single servings.

Single servings can be slightly more expensive, but in the long run you'll save both calories and money. How many times did you open a large bag of chips to have "just a few," and before you knew it the bag was empty? With a one-ounce bag of chips, you enjoy a favorite without sabotaging your weight loss goals. Single-serving pudding, ice cream, snack-size yogurt and pretzels, candy bars, and mini bags of peanuts will help keep your overindulging under control.

Small sizes = a smaller you.

There are no exceptions—order small-size sodas, movie theater popcorn, ice cream cones, fries, even enjoy small- to medium-size fresh fruits. Whenever you are tempted to order "grande," "super," or "jumbo," say to yourself, "Do *I* want to be 'grande,' 'super,' or 'jumbo'?"

On the side, measure, don't pour.

Butter, sour cream, sauce, gravy, mayonnaise, salad dressing, syrup, cocktail sauce, tartar sauce, and ketchup can add calories quickly. Spoon out a small serving and put the container away. Try dipping your empty fork into the "add-on" before you add a forkful of food, rather than dunking the food into the dressing or sauce. Fork-first adds taste but far less calories.

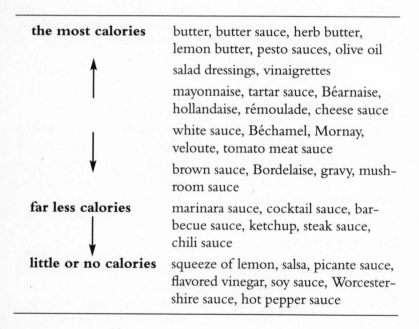

the most calories	butter, butter sauce, herb butter, lemon butter, pesto sauces, olive oil
↑	salad dressings, vinaigrettes
	mayonnaise, tartar sauce, Béarnaise, hollandaise, rémoulade, cheese sauce
↓	white sauce, Béchamel, Mornay, veloute, tomato meat sauce
	brown sauce, Bordelaise, gravy, mushroom sauce
far less calories	marinara sauce, cocktail sauce, barbecue sauce, ketchup, steak sauce, chili sauce
↓	
little or no calories	squeeze of lemon, salsa, picante sauce, flavored vinegar, soy sauce, Worcestershire sauce, hot pepper sauce

Chewing is satisfying.

Foods that require a lot of chewing slow down the eating process and give your brain time to recognize that you are satisfied. Try

Shredded Wheat, raw fruits and vegetables, vegetable-packed soups, fresh cherries, grapes, watermelon, pomegranates, steamed artichokes, unbuttered popcorn, and pretzels.

Go easy on calorie dense food.

Foods high in fat and sugar pack in more calories, bite for bite. While fats like butter, mayonnaise, salad dressing and sour cream can add calories on quickly, lowfat, high-sugar foods are also high in calories. Diets loaded with fruits, vegetables, and high-fiber breads and cereals help keep pounds off: diets filled with calorie-dense fried foods, cheese, candy, cake, cookies, and ice cream don't.

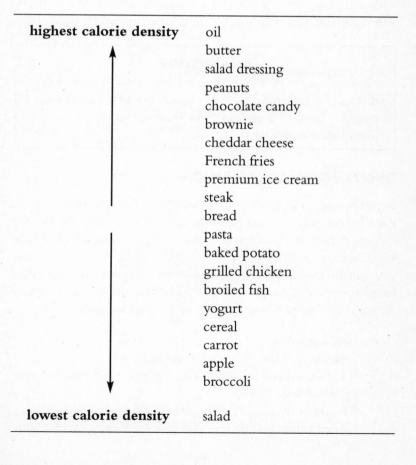

highest calorie density

oil
butter
salad dressing
peanuts
chocolate candy
brownie
cheddar cheese
French fries
premium ice cream
steak
bread
pasta
baked potato
grilled chicken
broiled fish
yogurt
cereal
carrot
apple
broccoli

lowest calorie density

salad

> ### SMART STUFF—A bite or a bowl?
> A two-ounce breaded chicken nugget has about 140 calories and offers you about two mouthfuls of food. A cup and a half of almost any soup (except creamed or cheese-topped) has the same calories but many more mouthfuls to enjoy.

Enjoy foods naked.

Whenever possible, undress your food to cut your calories. Baked potatoes without sour cream, vegetables without cheese sauce, bread without butter, meat without gravy, hamburgers without cheese, salads without dressing, ice cream without hot fudge, cake without icing—over a lifetime of healthy eating, these simple "dress-downs" can help you lose and maintain your weight.

> ### SMART STUFF
> Harvard researchers found that the three most important predictors of weight gain in middle-aged men were lack of exercise, too much time in front of the TV, and snacking on foods like cookies and chips.

Don't Feel Guilty About Eating Out

If you're going out to eat tonight don't worry—just make a plan. Eat a lighter breakfast and lunch in order to save a few calories for the larger portions you'll face this evening. It's not a bad idea to squeeze in some extra activity during the day as well. Or instead, you can balance tonight's meal with your choices and activities tomorrow. And there are lots of thin habits you can use to enjoy the evening without sabotaging your weight loss goals.

- *Avoid temptation.*
    Stay away from all-you-can-eat buffets.
    Take a roll and ask that the bread basket be removed from the table.
    Request no butter for the bread.
    Keep the vegetable tray and give back the chips and dip.

- *"Something to drink?"—"Water, thank you."*
    Choose calorie-free drinks—water, mineral water, club soda, unsweetened iced tea.
    Choose lower calorie drinks—wine, wine spritzers, fruit juice + club soda, diet soda.
- *Make an "appetizer" a meal.*
    Order an appetizer portion as an entrée.
    Ask if a luncheon portion can be ordered at dinner.
    Share a main dish and order extra vegetables.
- *Play with your food.*
    Scrape off extra sauce.
    Trim away excess fat.
    Remove skin from poultry.
    Remove butter or sour cream from the baked potato.
- *On the side.*
    Ask that butter, gravy, salad dressing, sauce, sour cream, syrup, guacamole, grated cheese, be served on the side.
- *Eat slowly.*
    Enjoy the company—talk more, eat less.
    Take in the ambience of the restaurant.
- *Eat until you feel fine, not full.*
    Stop eating when you feel comfortably satisfied, not stuffed.
    You don't have to clean your plate.
    Ask for a "doggie bag" to take home.
- *Split dessert.*
    Share with another person or, better yet, with the whole table.

SMART STUFF

According to a survey done by the American Institute for Cancer Research (AICR), 67% of Americans always or almost always finish their restaurant portions. Men are 4 times more likely than women to eat their entire entrée, even when the portion is too large. AICR cautions that eating out often, and unthinkingly eating all that extra food, contributes to obesity and obesity-related diseases.

Reinforce Thin Habits

One of our clients' favorite "take-home" reminders is the list of thin habits. We'll remind you to read these over often because we know it takes time and reinforcement to trade old habits for new good ones.

Get Skinny's *Thin Habits*

When to eat
- *Eat when you're hungry.*
- *Eat regular meals plus a snack or two.*
- *Eat breakfast.*
- *Skip the midnight feeding.*

How to eat
- *Eat slowly.*
- *Leave serving dishes on the counter or stove.*
- *Eat from plates, not packages.*
- *Eat at the table.*
- *Quit the "clean plate club."*
- *Resist the "Now I've blown it!" syndrome.*
- *Keep food out of sight, out of reach.*

What to eat
- *Start with soup.*
- *Eat more fruits and vegetables, drink less juice.*
- *Curb calories in a glass.*
- *Fat free doesn't equal calorie free.*
- *Fill up on fiber.*
- *Buy single servings.*
- *Small sizes = smaller you.*
- *On the side, measure, don't pour.*
- *Chew, it's satisfying.*
- *Go easy on calorie dense food.*
- *Enjoy foods naked.*

THE POWER OF PORTIONS

Obesity became an epidemic in this country at the same time that portion sizes grew enormous.

—American Institute for Cancer Research

The U.S. food supply produces enough food to supply approximately 3700 calories per person per day. Yet, in the third National Health and Nutrition Examination Survey (NHANES III), the average calorie intake reported by those surveyed was 2095 calories a day. A discrepancy of more than 1600 calories a day is too large to be due to plate waste (food served but not eaten). Experts theorize that this discrepancy is more likely due to people under-reporting the size of their portions.

That's easy to believe, because research has shown that people cannot evaluate portions accurately. And it is not the public's fault. The "typical" portion size often differs on food labels, in dietary guidelines, and in the amount of food you are served when you eat out. How can you be expected to reach your target calorie zone if you cannot accurately evaluate the portion sizes you are eating?

The *Get Skinny* diet is going to end your confusion once and for all. First, we are going to draw a distinction between a "serving" and a "portion." Then we'll give visual clues to help you estimate the size of the portion you are facing. Finally, we'll give you average calorie counts in "typical" portions. Armed with all this, you'll be able to determine the size of any portion of food and guesstimate the calories. If that isn't enough, in Appendix 3 you'll find a calorie counter for over 600 commonly eaten foods.

SMART STUFF

According to a recent survey, 80% of doctors and dietitians said the most important thing Americans could do to improve their diets was to reduce their portion sizes.

In this section you'll learn how to turn portions into a powerful weapon to help you reach your target weight. Never again will you fall victim to overeating because you thought the muffin you bought at the coffee shop was an "average-size" portion. Most bakery, deli, or coffee shop muffins are anything but average. As a matter of fact, some can weigh a quarter of a pound and have over 400 calories. That equals 4 average servings.

How did portion sizes get so out of control? Interestingly, no one gave much thought to portions before the 1950s and until very recently, little research was done regarding their impact on weight gain. As portion sizes increased, the variety of food eaten decreased, thereby cutting down on the intake of fiber and necessary nutrients. Eating large portions on a regular basis overrides the natural feeling of fullness and makes it all too easy for overeating to become a habit.

SMART STUFF—Commonsense portions can curb heartburn

Heartburn sufferers are often told to cut back on fatty foods, advice that may do more for your heart than your heartburn. A recent study published in the *European Journal of Gastroenterology and Hepatology* showed that it wasn't the greasy foods but eating too much at one time that caused the problem.

In 1958 the USDA issued its first public health eating guide, the "Basic Four," which divided foods into 4 main categories and provided recommendations for the size of a serving and the number of servings to be eaten daily. There was no research done to define a "serving." Instead, the amount of food recommended was based on the 1953 version of the Recommended Dietary Allowances (RDA), which gave calorie and nutrient intakes for healthy people. For example, a 2- to 3-ounce portion of meat provided half the RDA for protein. A half-cup portion of citrus fruit met the RDA for vitamin C, and so on. Almost fifty years later most of these early portion recommendations, though antiquated, are still commonly used.

In 1992, the government released the Food Guide Pyramid, the first visual guide for how much and what to eat daily. While, in concept, the pyramid is excellent, it can often be confusing in practice. For example, the vegetable, fruit, and bread and grain groups offer suggested portions for the day: 3 to 5 vegetables, 2 to

4 fruits, and 6 to 11 breads or other grain foods. The meat and dairy groups, in contrast, base their portions on equivalents: how much protein is available from a portion of meat, fish, beans, nuts or eggs; how much cheese or yogurt you have to eat to equal the same amount of calcium in one glass of milk. Also, National Education and Labeling Act (NELA), passed by Congress in 1990, legally defined uniform serving sizes for use on food labels. These serving sizes were developed based on consumption surveys done in the 1980s and resulted in servings that were often larger than those used in the Food Guide Pyramid.

Considering all this, it's no wonder you and the rest of the American public are confused! The government is offering conflicting standards for an "average" serving while you are faced with bagel, soda, sandwich, and pasta servings that are getting larger by the minute. The *Get Skinny* diet is about to replace this confusion with common sense.

Let's start by defining the difference between a "serving" and a "portion." A **serving is a standard measurement of food.** For example, the Food Guide Pyramid tells you that a serving of pasta is a half cup. A **portion is the amount of food you are served.** A typical restaurant portion of pasta equals 3 cups, which translates into 6 servings, according to the Food Guide Pyramid. We'd like to put an end to this silly comparison and necessary conversion by declaring that a portion and a serving equal the same thing—a reasonable amount of food. We'll then add to this the number of calories found in a "commonsense" portion.

Get Skinny's Commonsense Portions

Carbohydrate Foods

Let's begin with bread and foods high in carbohydrate, because this is a very misunderstood group. Some tell you carbohydrates make you fat, others recommend that foods high in carbohydrate should be the foundation of your diet. Who's right? Both, to some degree.

Carbohydrate foods that are high in fiber and low in sugar, like brown rice and whole wheat bread, pasta and cereal, do help you lose weight. They are satisfying to chew and their fiber content increases your feeling of fullness and satisfaction without adding calories. More calorie dense carbohydrate foods like white rice, regular pasta, pancakes, muffins, and bagels offer no fiber and some experts suggest that these foods promote overeating.

We'd encourage including more whole grain carbohydrate choices but we are not opposed to any carbohydrate foods in particular. The key, we believe, is awareness of calorie density and control of portion sizes. The following table, *Get Skinny*'s Commonsense Portions: Bread, Cereal, Pasta, Rice, Beans and other Carbohydrate-Dense Foods, clearly illustrates this. A slice of bread—a commonsense portion—has about 100 calories. So does a cup of most varieties of dry cereal.

But when was the last time you ate one cup of pasta and happily declared that dinner? Not lately, would be our guess. Typically we eat at least two and, more often, three cups of pasta as a serving. We are not suggesting you eat just one cup of pasta. The point we are making is that you need to be able to evaluate how much pasta is on the plate so that you will not underestimate the portion and the number of calories, a typical mistake most people make.

A commonsense portion of cooked cereal, rice, and beans is one cup. But you can see from the chart that these choices are more calorie dense, so one portion provides more calories.

Get Skinny's Commonsense Portions: Bread, Cereal, Pasta, Rice, Beans and Other Carbohydrate-Dense Foods

Food	Commonsense Portion	Calories Per Portion
Bread	1 slice	100
Cereal, dry	1 cup	100
Popcorn, unbuttered	2 cups	100
Toaster waffle	1, 4-inch square	100
Cereal, cooked	1 cup	150
Pancake	1, 6-inch diameter	150
Rice, cooked	1 cup	200
Beans	1 cup	200
Pasta, cooked	2 cups	400

This guide is useful to a point but there are many carbohydrate-rich foods that don't neatly fit into this group. What about a bagel? Muffin? Roll? Large soft pretzel? Here is where you switch to a visual cue. A yo-yo is the same size as a mini-bagel, which weighs 1 ounce and has about 100 calories. Now take that same yo-yo size and place it next to a typical bagel from a bagel store. The bagel store bagel will easily equal 2 and maybe 3 yo-yos. If it equals 3 yo-yos, it's 3 ounces and equals 300 calories; 5 yo-yos equals 5 ounces and 500 calories. You're probably beginning to see how easy it is to overeat while at the same time underestimating your intake.

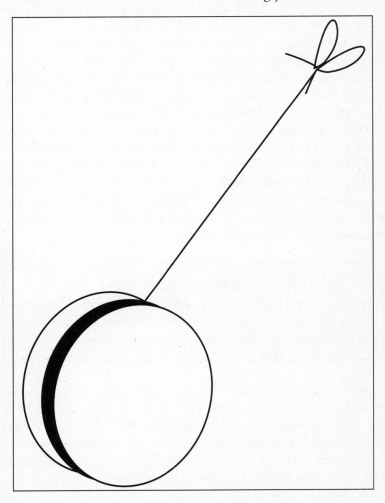

You can use the yo-yo equivalent to "guesstimate" the calories of many other choices—the roll on your lunch sandwich, the muffin you have with coffee, a doughnut, a Belgian waffle. Though not foolproof, it is a good tool to help you visualize the size of the portions you eat.

Protein Choices

When you are trying to lose weight, the second most problematic group of foods are those high in protein. A commonsense portion of meat, fish or poultry is 4 ounces. A restaurant serving can often be double or triple that amount. A 4-ounce serving of boneless meat, fish or poultry is about the size of a computer mouse, one-half inch thick (the thickness of the mouse end). *Get Skinny's* Commonsense Portions: Meat, Fish and Poultry, gives the approximate calories in a 4-ounce serving of different protein choices. The calories per portion go up as the fat content goes up.

Now that you can accurately estimate a 4-ounce commonsense portion of protein, consider making smaller portions when you cook at home. When eating out, think about splitting an entrée with a friend or bringing home some in a doggie bag. If, on occasion, you decide to eat a larger portion, that's okay, as long as you correctly estimate the portion and accurately keep track of the calories you've eaten.

SMART STUFF

Another visual clue to help you keep protein portions in check is to fill ¾ of your dinner plate with vegetables, fruits, and grains and ¼ with meat, fish or poultry (the protein choice).

When we suggested the doggie bag tip to one of our clients, he said, "If I order a Big Mac, I'm not going to eat half and tote the rest of it around in my briefcase all day." We agree. Instead we suggested a single hamburger—a commonsense portion. Remember, when it comes to eating you are always in charge. Use your common sense to make a compromise and save calories.

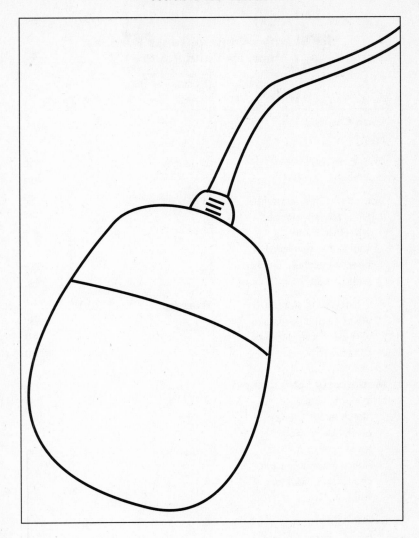

Fruits and Vegetables

Anytime you're hungry, anytime you have an urge to eat that is hard to control, think fruits and vegetables. Although the entire focus of *Your Personalized Weight Attack Plan* is to get you to tune in to your body's signals and learn how to accurately estimate how much you eat, you probably aren't eating enough fruits and vegetables. Very few people do.

Get Skinny's Commonsense Portions: Meat, Fish and Poultry

Food	Commonsense Portion	Calories Per Portion
Lean Choices		
Egg		100
Cod, crab, pollack, scallops, scrod	4 ounces	120
Abalone, clams, lobster, tuna, shrimp, smoked whitefish, oysters, shark, lox, deli roast beef, white meat chicken without skin, ham, halibut	4 ounces	160
Pork tenderloin, salmon, white meat chicken with skin, roast turkey breast without skin	4 ounces	200
Moderately Lean Choices		
Strip steak, veal, filet mignon, London broil, beef kabobs, roast beef, pot roast, stir-fry meat, loin pork chop, dark meat turkey without skin, tuna in oil	4 ounces	240
Sirloin steak, rib steak, brisket, corned beef, T-bone steak, fajitas, leg of lamb, dark meat chicken with skin, chicken fingers	4 ounces	280

Food	Commonsense Portion	Calories Per Portion
Higher Fat Choices		
Porterhouse steak, pork spareribs, fried clams and oysters, fried dark meat chicken, hamburger	4 ounces	320
Sausage, lamb chops, prime rib, fried fish, fried chicken wings, salami, bologna, pastrami, meatloaf	4 ounces	400
Tuna salad	4 ounces (about 1 cup)	400
Egg salad	4 ounces (about 1 cup)	600

Aside from French fries, most Americans barely eat two servings of fruits and vegetables a day. Five servings would be a much healthier goal. If you skip the fried varieties and take off the butter and cheese sauce, vegetables, as a group, are a pretty low-calorie bunch. Medium-size fruits are excellent choices as well. Both fruits and vegetables are low in calories and rich in vitamins, minerals, antioxidants and fiber.

We've recommended, as a thin habit, that until you reach your target weight you have *more fruits and vegetables, less juice.* That's simply because juice is more calorie dense, it eliminates the satisfaction of chewing and it has little of the fiber found in the whole fruit or vegetable.

Once again you can see that plain vegetables and fresh fruit are less calorie dense. The way vegetables are cooked or the addition of syrup to canned fruit adds more calories. Starchy vegetables,

Get Skinny's Commonsense Portions: Fruits and Vegetables

Food	Commonsense Portion	Calories Per Portion
Vegetables,* steamed	1 cup	50
Fruit,** fresh	1 cup or 1 medium	70
Vegetables, stewed (ratatouille, stewed tomatoes)	1 cup	75
Fruit salad or canned fruit, light syrup	1 cup	100
Vegetables,* stir-fried	1 cup	100
Tossed salad without dressing	2 cups	100
Fruit juice	1 cup	120
Corn on the cob	1, 6-inch ear	150
Potato, corn, peas, plantain, sweet potato, winter squash	1 cup	150
Potato, baked	1 medium (6 ounces)	200

*asparagus, bamboo shoots, bean sprouts, broccoli, Brussels sprouts, cabbage, carrots, cauliflower, celery, cucumber, eggplant, green beans, greens, kohlrabi, leeks, mushrooms, okra, onions, peapods, peppers, sauerkraut, spinach, tomatoes, water chestnuts, wax beans, yellow squash, zucchini

**apple, apricot, banana, blueberries, cherries, grapefruit, grapes, kiwi, mango, melon, nectarine, orange, papaya, peach, pear, pineapple, plum, raspberries, strawberries, tangerine, watermelon

like potatoes, corn, and winter squash, though healthy choices, are also more calorie dense. To estimate calories accurately, you need to be aware of this.

You can use two visual clues to help you estimate portion sizes: a tennis ball equals a medium fresh fruit and a computer mouse equals a medium baked potato.

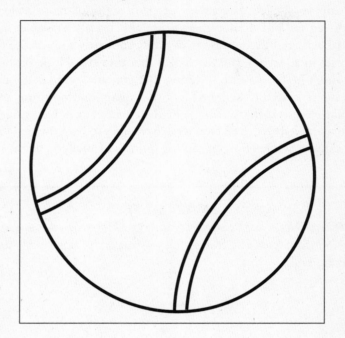

Milk, Cheese, Yogurt and Ice Cream

In order to reduce calories, many of our clients cut out this group of foods. The easiest way to cut calories and still get all the essential nutrients found in this group, like calcium, is to choose nonfat or lowfat varieties. Whole milk, cheese, yogurt and ice cream are more calorie dense.

Many of our clients find it hard to jump from drinking regular whole milk to nonfat milk. Do it in stages: this week buy 2% milk, next 1% and finally nonfat. If you enjoy cream in your coffee, use whole milk or evaporated lowfat or nonfat milk for a creamy taste.

The flavor of cheese goes a long way. Instead of chunks or slices use grated or shredded cheese. You can even top a sandwich with shredded cheese. By doing so, you'll still get the flavor with far less calories. A teaspoon of cheese that delivers a punch of flavor, like feta, blue cheese, extra sharp cheddar, or parmesan, can add zip to a salad, vegetables or pasta without many calories. Reduced fat and nonfat cheeses are also readily available. Read the labels carefully because many only modestly reduce the total calories in a serving. But that's okay, because every little bit helps. Just don't be fooled into thinking that you are saving many calories by making this switch. The other disappointing thing about nonfat cheese is that it does not melt well. Consider using half nonfat and half reduced fat cheese in recipes to reap the benefit of less calories while enjoying the creaminess of melted cheese.

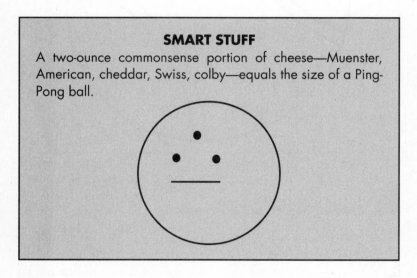

SMART STUFF
A two-ounce commonsense portion of cheese—Muenster, American, cheddar, Swiss, colby—equals the size of a Ping-Pong ball.

Reduced fat or fat free cottage cheese and ricotta cheese can help you save calories and are versatile for breakfast, lunch, dinner or dessert. Spread some on an English muffin for breakfast instead of cream cheese. Use as the base for a luncheon fruit salad. Mix a small amount of ricotta with tomato sauce for a creamy but not too rich pasta sauce. Make a healthy cheese danish by toasting a slice of raisin bread, spreading it with cottage cheese, and sprinkling cinnamon sugar on top.

> **SMART STUFF—A commonsense dish**
> A serving of ice cream is not a soup bowl full! Find a small
> dish in your kitchen that holds about a half-cup and call it the
> "commonsense ice cream dish."

Premium ice cream has almost twice the calories of reduced fat
varieties. Nonfat ice cream is a good choice, too, but it may not
be much lower in calories than reduced fat flavors. All too often
the nonfat choices contain a good deal of added sugar, so the
overall calorie reduction is not as much as you would think. Look
for reduced fat and nonfat frozen yogurt. On the *Get Skinny*'s
Commonsense Portions: Milk, Cheese, Yogurt, Ice Cream, we
have compared only vanilla-flavored ice cream because other flavors and the addition of chips, nuts, fruit, marshmallows, etc. vary
so widely in calories that it is not possible to come up with an
"average." When you select a brand and flavor of your choice,
read the label and track your calories accurately. The best way to
deal with ice cream is to eat only a commonsense half-cup portion or avoid temptation by buying single-serving varieties, like
Dixie cups and pops.

> **SMART STUFF—Feel like an ice cream cone?**
> Don't take the cone for granted. A regular, wafer-type cone
> has 17 calories, a sugar cone 40 and a large waffle cone,
> 120 calories.

There are hundreds of yogurts to pick from out there. Some
brands offer a staggering array of choices—regular (made with
whole milk), lowfat or nonfat, and light (artificially sweetened)—
all with an endless variety of flavors. The best yogurt choice is
nonfat plain. Flavors, fruits and toppings add extra calories. You
can top plain yogurt with crunchy dry cereal or fresh fruit. Consider keeping snack-size lowfat or nonfat yogurts on hand as a

Get Skinny's **Commonsense Portions: Milk, Cheese, Yogurt, Ice Cream**

Food	Commonsense Portion	Calories Per Portion
Milk, regular or whole	1 cup	150
Milk, 2%	1 cup	120
Milk, 1%	1 cup	100
Nonfat milk, buttermilk	1 cup	80
Yogurt, nonfat flavored[1]	8 ounces (1 container)	150
Yogurt, snack-size	4 ounces (1 container)	120
Yogurt, nonfat plain[2]	8 ounces (1 container)	120
Ice cream, rich or premium vanilla[3]	½ cup	170
Ice cream, reduced fat vanilla[4]	½ cup	110
Ice cream, nonfat vanilla[5]	½ cup	90
Frozen yogurt, vanilla[6]	½ cup	115
Cheese[7]	2 ounces	220
Cottage cheese, nonfat[8]	½ cup	80
Ricotta cheese, nonfat[9]	½ cup	110

[1]Calories are based on averages from brands currently available, which vary from 70 to 210 calories in an 8-ounce container.

[2]Calories are based on averages from brands currently available, which vary from 110 to 130 calories in an 8-ounce container.

[3]Calories are based on averages from brands currently available, which vary from 130 to 270 calories in a half-cup portion.

[4]Calories are based on averages from brands currently available, which vary from 92 to 130 calories in a half-cup portion.

[5]Calories are based on averages from brands currently available, which vary from 80 to 100 calories in a half-cup portion.

[6]Calories are based on averages from brands currently available, which vary from 80 to 140 calories in a half-cup portion.

[7]Reduced-fat and nonfat cheese will have less calories per portion.

[8]Calories are based on averages from brands currently available, which vary from 70 to 90 calories in a half-cup portion.

[9]Calories are based on averages from brands currently available, which vary from 100 to 120 calories in a half-cup portion.

moderate calorie, between-meal treat. *Get Skinny*'s Commonsense Portions gives you calorie values for nonfat plain yogurt and flavored nonfat yogurt. These values are based on averages from yogurt brands currently available. Whatever brand of yogurt you buy, read the label carefully, as calorie values for the same size container can vary enormously. For example, flavored yogurt labeled "lowfat," "fat free" or "light" can have anywhere from 90 to 240 calories in an eight-ounce container.

Cheese, ice cream, frozen yogurt and yogurt brands continually change as companies market new flavors and varieties. Use *Get Skinny*'s Commonsense Portions but also check the label of your favorite brand to be sure you are accurately targeting your calorie zone.

When you drink a glass of milk, just how big a portion are you having? The drawing of an 8-ounce glass on the next page may surprise you. It is probably smaller than you imagined and is most likely smaller than the glass you regularly use at home. To be sure you are not underestimating a "glassful," measure your glasses by filling them with water and pouring the water into a measuring cup. Most household drinking glasses hold 10, 12 or even 15 ounces. Filling up a large glass may actually equal two commonsense portions.

SMART STUFF

To help you accurately track calories, use a 1 cup measuring cup as a pitcher to pour milk over cereal. This way you can accurately tell how much you've added.

Calories count and commonsense portions help you cut calories. You can lose a pound by cutting 3500 calories. It's easier than you think. The following chart offers some easy changes you can make.

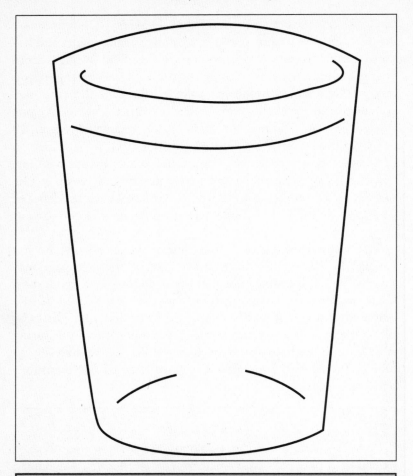

SMART STUFF—Practice portions

Research has shown that pictures and food models do not help people recognize portion amounts. But practice works. Practice portions by measuring out the Commonsense Portions and putting them on your dishes. By doing this repeatedly, when you first start your weight loss program, you will teach yourself to visualize commonsense portions of food.

What does a cup of rice look like? Two cups of pasta? A cup of dry cereal—surprised to find it doesn't fill the bowl? But 2 cups of salad is probably more than you thought. Keep practicing!

Cutting Calories
1 Pound = 3500 Calories

Typical Serving	Get Skinny's Commonsense Portion	Calories Cut
Movie theater popcorn, small, 7 cups **400 calories**	Popcorn, unbuttered 2 cups **100 calories**	**300**
24-hour store, Double Gulp soda, 8 cups (64 ounces) **800 calories**	1 can soda, 12 ounces **140 calories**	**660**
Medium coffee + 2 tablespoons half & half, 2 teaspoons sugar **120 calories**	Small coffee + 2 tablespoons skim milk, 1 teaspoon sugar **26 calories**	**94**
Restaurant serving tuna salad, 8 ounces **800 calories**	Tuna salad, 4 ounces **400 calories**	**400**
Salad with 2 tablespoons creamy Italian dressing **320 calories**	Salad with 2 tablespoons fat free creamy Italian dressing **200 calories**	**120**
Restaurant serving pasta, 3 cups **600 calories**	Cooked pasta, any shape, 2 cups **400 calories**	**200**
Steakhouse 1 pound porterhouse steak cooked, 17 ounces **1190 calories**	Steakhouse 8-ounce boneless sirloin cooked, 7 ounces **420 calories**	**770**
Baked potato + ¼ cup sour cream **320 calories**	Baked potato + freshly ground pepper **200 calories**	**120**
Pancake House Pancakes (4) **800 calories**	Pancake House Short Stack (2) **400 calories**	**400**

(continued)

	Cutting Calories (cont.) **1 Pound = 3500 Calories**	
Typical Serving	Get Skinny's Commonsense Portion	Calories Cut
1 cup cereal + 1 cup whole milk **260 calories**	1 cup cereal + 1 cup nonfat milk **180 calories**	**80**
Ice cream cone 1 cup premium vanilla in sugar cone **380 calories**	Ice cream cone 1 cup frozen yogurt vanilla in wafer cone **197 calories**	**183**
Carrot cake with cream cheese frosting **484 calories**	Carrot cake with cream cheese frosting split with a friend **242 calories**	**242**
Total Calories Saved		**3569 calories—** **more than** **1 pound**

Add-ons Add Up

Though we've encouraged you to *enjoy foods naked,* we appreciate that there are times when we all need to dress our foods. Sweet and fatty additions can add on calories quicker than you realize.

Over the last ten years there has been a big emphasis on cutting out or cutting down the fat in your diet. Americans have modestly reduced their total fat intake and have made a shift away from saturated fats toward more polyunsaturated and mono-unsaturated fats. That's the good news. The bad news is that at the same time Americans have increased the amount of sugar they eat, creating a net gain of over 100 calories per person per day.

We're not against eating some sugar. For that matter, we're not against eating some fat. But you've read enough so far to realize that you need to keep your intake of fats and sweets moderate and you need to carefully track the calories they contribute.

SMART STUFF

Research has shown that American adults eat one-third of their day's calories as energy-dense, nutrient-poor foods—butter, margarine, oils, salad dressings, gravies, sugar, sweeteners, desserts and salty snacks.

Fats

Mist instead of pour.

Measure instead of pour.

Foods high in fat are very calorie dense. Pure fats have the highest calorie density. Adding just a little butter, sour cream, salad dressing, mayonnaise or oil to a food can make calories soar. Misting and measuring are two simple, easy steps to keep fat calories down.

Get Skinny's Commonsense Portions: Foods High in Fat

Food	Commonsense Portion	Calories Per Portion
Oil olive, corn, canola[1]	1 tablespoon	120
Butter	1 tablespoon	100
Whipped butter	1 tablespoon	80
Cream cheese[2]	2 tablespoons	100
Whipped cream cheese	2 tablespoons	70
Half & Half	2 tablespoons	80
Lard or vegetable shortening	1 tablespoon	115
Margarine[3]	1 tablespoon	100

(continued)

Get Skinny's **Commonsense Portions: Foods High in Fat (cont.)**

Food	Commonsense Portion	Calories Per Portion
Whipped or tub margarine	1 tablespoon	60
Mayonnaise[4]	1 tablespoon	110
Peanut butter[5]	2 tablespoons	190
Salad dressing, all flavors[6]	2 tablespoons	130
Reduced fat salad dressing, all flavors[7]	2 tablespoons	100
Sour cream[8]	2 tablespoons	60
Nonfat sour cream[9]	2 tablespoons	25
Tartar sauce	2 tablespoons	150
Whipped cream	¼ cup	100

[1]All varieties of vegetable oil have 120 calories in a tablespoon.

[2]Cream cheese brands can be found fat free, light and flavored. Some choices reduce calories slightly while others add some. Read labels carefully.

[3]Some brands of margarine have light or reduced fat varieties, which will reduce calories somewhat. Read labels carefully.

[4]Some brands of mayonnaise have light or reduced fat varieties, which will reduce calories somewhat. Read labels carefully.

[5]Some brands of peanut butter have light or reduced fat varieties, which will reduce calories somewhat. Read labels carefully.

[6]Calories are based on averages from brands currently available, which vary from 90 to 180 calories in a 2-tablespoon portion.

[7]Calories are based on averages from brands currently available, which vary from 13 to 80 calories in a 2-tablespoon portion.

[8]Some brands of sour cream have a reduced fat variety with calories per portion falling somewhere between regular sour cream and nonfat sour cream.

[9]Calories are based on averages from brands currently available, which vary from 15 to 35 calories in a 2-tablespoon portion.

When cooking, use nonfat cooking spray to coat pans for frying. Many brands offer butter or olive oil varieties that can be used to add flavor to pasta, rice or vegetables without adding extra calories. Lightly spray after cooking to punch flavor but keep calories low. You can also make your own flavored oil by adding herbs to oil in a mister or spray bottle. Herb infused oil and vinegar misted on salads or cooked vegetables creates fuller flavor with a fraction of the calories.

When you can't mist, measure. Don't just pour oil into a frying pan, measure out a teaspoon or two. Use a tablespoon to portion out your salad dressing, sour cream, cream cheese or peanut butter. If you do this consistently you will save thousands of calories in a year, translating into weight loss and weight maintenance.

Another calorie saving tip is to use whipped and reduced-fat versions when possible. Most salad dressings, sour creams, Half & Half, and cream cheeses are available in reduced-fat and nonfat varieties. Though they will save some calories, none are calorie free. Read the labels of the brands you've chosen, measure the portion you're using, and track calories carefully. Whipped cream cheese, butter and margarine incorporate air into the food so that a serving has less calories than the more solid variety. While this is another way to save calories, it is not enough to give you license to eat any of these foods in unlimited amounts.

SMART STUFF—Add-ons that don't add up

Horseradish, hot sauce, canned au jus gravy, lemon juice, mustard, picante, salsa, soy sauce, vinegar, and Worcestershire sauce have so few calories that you can add them without adding on calories.

Salad dressings, like yogurt and ice cream, come in a mind-boggling number of varieties—regular, creamy, light, lowfat, nonfat, reduced fat—and in more flavors than one can imagine. It is hard to make generalizations about which to choose, but we can recommend that you use a commonsense portion and read the label carefully so that you track calories accurately. One thing you can be sure of though, no brand is calorie free! The label of your favorite brand will be your best guide.

Sugar and Other Sweet Add-ons

In the last 15 years per capita consumption of sugar rose a whopping 28%, to 53 teaspoons a day. Experts recommend only 10 teaspoons a day. Unfortunately, wherever you turn there is something sweet to entice you: sweetened cereal, sweetened fruit drinks, cookies, candy, cake, pastries, and more. Though not as calorie dense as fat, sugar has calories and when you eat a lot it adds up to extra weight. We are not suggesting that you cut out sugar but like all our other advice, we want you to use common-sense portions and track calories carefully.

SMART STUFF—"Just coffee, thank you."

Unless you order "black, no sugar," the calories add up.
Coffee or tea with cream and sugar = 10 calories an ounce.

1 small coffee (10 ounces) = 100 calories
1 medium coffee (12 ounces) = 120 calories
1 large coffee (16 ounces) = 160 calories

Why didn't we suggest using artificial sweeteners and artificially sweetened foods to cut calories? We have nothing against using these, but they don't keep you from gaining weight. As Americans get fatter and fatter, it has never been proven that using sweeteners actually helps weight loss. In fact, some research has shown that we eat the same amount of calories whether sweeteners are used or not, perhaps because we are trying to make up for the calorie deficit.

SMART STUFF

A handy visual clue to estimate one teaspoon is the approximate size of your thumbnail.

Get Skinny's Commonsense Portions: Sugar and Other Sweet Add-ons

Food	Commonsense Portion	Calories Per Portion
Pancake syrup	2 tablespoons	120
Chocolate syrup	2 tablespoons	100
Jelly, jam	1 tablespoon	50
All fruit jelly	1 tablespoon	35
Honey	1 teaspoon	20
Brown sugar	1 teaspoon	15
Sugar	1 teaspoon	15
Powdered sugar	1 teaspoon	10

One of our clients once reported having a calorie-laden lunch with a diet soda. When we questioned the choice of the diet soda, she said laughingly, "It's my token offering to the diet god." This offhand remark holds a lot of truth—using an artificial sweetener only makes a token dent in your total calorie intake. If you want to use sweeteners, that's fine, but be realistic about their true contribution to your weight loss plan.

SMART STUFF

Even with the availability of diet soda, 80% of all the soda we drink is sweetened. It's been estimated that the average American drinks 41 gallons of sweetened soda a year or 1.2 cans a day. That could equal a 20-pound weight gain in a year.

A Word About Alcohol

Most experts are in agreement—a moderate amount of alcohol has health benefits. But while you are counting up your health benefits, you also need to be counting calories. The calories in alcohol, though not as well utilized by the body as food calories, do add up.

Sweet after-dinner cordials average 100 calories an ounce (a two-ounce serving is the norm); hard liquor averages 80 calories an ounce (a typical shot glass is 1½ ounces); wine averages 25 calories an ounce (most wineglasses hold a minimum of 5 ounces and often much more); beer averages 12 calories an ounce and light beer 9 (a large draft glass can hold a pint, or 16 ounces). Mixed drinks like piña colada, Irish coffee or a Long Island iced tea can easily be 250 calories or more.

Reinforce Commonsense Portions

Bread, cereal, pasta, rice, beans and other carbohydrate-dense foods	pages 64–65
Meat, fish, poultry	pages 68–69
Fruits and Vegetables	page 70
Milk, cheese, yogurt, ice cream	page 74
Foods high in fat	pages 79–80
Sugar and other sweet add-ons	page 83

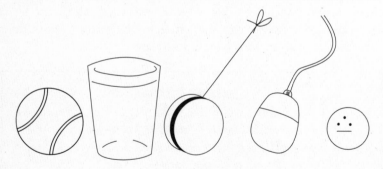

Reinforce Visual Clues to Estimate Commonsense Portions

Carbohydrate foods:	
Yo-yo	Equals one ounce or 100 calories
Protein foods:	
Computer mouse	Equals a four-ounce portion of meat, fish, or poultry

Fruit:	
Tennis ball	Equals a medium fruit
Potato:	
Computer mouse	Equals a medium baked potato
Cheese:	
Ping-Pong ball	Equals a two-ounce portion of cheese

SMART STUFF—Don't lose your common sense.
Research shows that regardless of how hungry you are, people eat more when presented with large portions of food. Simply knowing this can prevent you from overeating.

EXERCISE = ENJOYMENT

Each year, 250,000 deaths reported in the U.S. are attributed to physical inactivity. Not exercising is as dangerous as smoking, obesity, hypertension and drunken driving.
—Centers for Disease Control and Prevention

Activity speeds up your metabolism so that you can burn more calories faster. You don't need to run a marathon or be slumped over a Stairmaster after a workout to benefit from exercise. "Just get off your seat and on your feet." says former Surgeon General C. Everett Koop. Koop's philosophy is reinforced by the American College of Sports Medicine (ACSM), the American Heart Association (AHA) and the Centers for Disease Control and Prevention (CDC)—they all recommend that every adult get 30 minutes of physical activity on most and preferably all days of the week.

Recent studies show that activity not only burns calories and helps you lose weight, but it might save your life as well. Exercise dramatically lowers your risk for heart disease, it strengthens the immune system, promotes mental health, and reduces the risk of developing diabetes, osteoporosis and some cancers. It can give you a better outlook on life by fighting depression, releasing tension, increasing sexual desire and helping you think more clearly. Regular exercise relieves many symptoms of PMS (premenstrual syndrome) and menopause. Exercising cannot guarantee that you'll never have health problems just as buckling your seat belt cannot guarantee you'll never be hurt in a car accident. But regularly doing both significantly reduces your risk.

Proven Benefits of Exercise

Research shows that exercise:

- Helps you lose weight
- Helps to control weight
- Decreases the proportion of body fat and increases the amount of muscle
- Increases energy
- Reduces the risk of dying prematurely
- Reduces the risk of dying from heart disease
- Increases HDL, or "good" cholesterol
- Lowers LDL, or "bad" cholesterol
- Lowers triglyceride levels
- Reduces the risk of developing diabetes
- Helps to reduce blood sugar levels in people with diabetes
- Reduces the risk of developing high blood pressure
- Reduces blood pressure in people with high blood pressure
- Keeps blood pressure lower when you are stressed
- Reduces the risk of gallstones
- Reduces the risk of colon, breast, lung and prostate cancer
- Bolsters your immune system, reducing the incidence of colds and infections
- Helps to control depression and anxiety
- Helps to build and maintain strong bones, muscles and joints
- Helps to prevent and treat osteoporosis
- Improves sleep
- Promotes healthy, active aging
- Relieves arthritis
- Promotes psychological well-being

We know what you're thinking, we've heard it all before from our clients. You're too busy to go to the gym. You don't have enough stamina to take an exercise class. You haven't exercised in years. You're uncoordinated and were never good at sports.

We're going to give you the easiest exercise program ever—**just move!** We'll encourage you—as we encourage all our clients—to get involved in an exercise program that incorporates flexibility, strength and aerobics (cardiovascular endurance). Some people love the gym and find formal classes at scheduled times the best way to stay fit. But the great news is that you can accomplish all this and never enter a gym.

SMART STUFF—Exercise makes you sexy

After reviewing a number of studies, the American Council on Exercise concluded that regular, moderate exercise may help prevent, reduce or even reverse major sexual problems, including erectile dysfunction and low sex drive in men and women. Middle-aged men who burn 200 calories a day exercising cut their risk of impotence in half.

A two-year study by the Cooper Institute of Aerobics Research in Dallas, a nationally recognized fitness center, showed that many simple lifestyle changes offered the same benefits as a structured workout program. Those who made these lifestyle changes kept track of their activity every day. They walked stairs instead of taking escalators, cleaned the house, did yard work, started a walking program. In short, they **moved,** as often and as much as they could throughout the day.

To get you moving, let's look at what you can gain from 10 minutes of activity a day. Ten minutes of lying on the couch watching TV burns about 15 calories.* If you simply sit up, you'll burn 20 calories. Getting the picture? Walking in place for 10 minutes burns 40 calories; jogging bumps you to 90. Are you motivated yet? Just adding a leisurely 10-minute walk a day to

*Calculations based on a 150-pound person

your normal routine can burn 14,600 calories a year! And burning calories is only part of the story.

SMART STUFF—Don't sit your life away
Americans average 23 hours a week in front of the TV. That equals almost one day a week, adding up to 10 years over an average lifetime!

Today we use 400 fewer calories a day than our slimmer ancestors at the turn of the twentieth century. We have systematically engineered activity out of our lives, to the point where we don't even need to get up to change TV channels or get out of the car to open the garage door. The math is simple: take in an extra 100 calories a day (the amount in 1 slice of bread), multiply that by 365 days in a year and the result is a gain of about 10 pounds! Reverse this equation and use up an extra 100 calories a day through activity and you'd lose 10 pounds!

Just adding more activity to your day may not give you a six-pack midriff or a *Baywatch* body, but it will tone parts you can't see like your heart and lungs. All day, every day, there are opportunities for you to be more active. And on any given day it is an easy way to use up hundreds of calories.

Real-Life Fitness

- Pace while you're talking on the phone.
- Deliver memos and messages in person rather than by e-mail or phone.
- Go window shopping.
- Clean your house—washing floors, vacuuming carpets, washing windows and scrubbing bathrooms equals vigorous exercise.
- Garden—weeding, hoeing, cutting the lawn, raking and trimming bushes burns as many calories as a game of tennis.
- Turn your lunch break into an exercise excursion.

- Carry a basket when shopping for a few items—it's like a free weight that keeps getting heavier and heavier; switch arms for a maximum workout.
- Sign up for a charity walk, bike or run.
- Turn off the TV one night a week and plan something active.
- Make exercise a hobby—take golf, tennis or skating lessons.
- Park your car at the farthest end of the parking lot.
- Take the stairs—you burn 10 calories for every flight you climb; over a lifetime that uses up thousands of calories.
- Dance—salsa, polka, tango—square dancers can cover 5 miles in an evening.
- Grocery shop—push, lift, bend—one hour in the supermarket burns as many calories as a half hour on the treadmill.
- Spend rainy weekend afternoons walking around a museum; when the sun shines go to the zoo.
- Wash the car.
- Go bowling instead of going to the movies.
- Walk the dog.
- Push the baby in a carriage; take the kids to the playground.
- Be an active spectator; walk the circumference of the soccer field while the kids are playing.
- Play games as a family—badminton, volleyball, stickball, croquet.

SMART STUFF—Every trip counts!

Researchers at the University of Ulster in Belfast found that women who climbed stairs for as little as two minutes a day had lower cholesterol levels and improved resting pulse rates.

Getting Started

Sometimes the biggest obstacle to starting an exercise program is the commitment to do it. You're not alone. According to the *Surgeon General's Report on Physical Activity and Health,* 25% of American adults are inactive, 53% are somewhat active but not active enough to gain health benefits, and a meager 22% get enough physical activity.

We are so committed to the need for exercise in a weight loss program that this part of *Your Personalized Weight Attack Plan* is not negotiable. Daily activity is a must! When all you do is cut calories, your body reacts as if it's starving, shifting into low gear to conserve energy; in short, you burn fewer calories, making it harder to lose weight. This is also the reason dieters frequently regain all the weight they've lost.

Add exercise and the whole picture changes. Exercise not only burns calories through activity but it also uses up fat tissue and promotes the building of lean muscle tissue. Muscles are 70 times as "metabolically active" as fat. This means a pound of muscle uses up 70 times more calories than a pound of fat. In other words, the more muscle (lean body tissue) you have the more calories you burn, pound for pound. The more fat you have the less calories you need. Instead of having your body's calorie burning mechanism shift into low gear as it does on low calorie diets, exercise shifts your body into high gear and uses up more calories. Regular activity and a diet planned to meet your target calorie zone is critical to permanent weight loss.

A good example of this theory in action is the National Weight Control Registry, which tracks people who successfully lost weight and kept it off. Of 3,000 registrants who lost an average of 60 pounds each and kept it off for 6 years, almost 100% of them used diet plus exercise to lose weight, and 95% used the same combination to maintain their loss. Many of these people had family histories of obesity and had been overweight since childhood, yet they were able to succeed.

Often our clients ask us, "If exercise is so important, why hasn't my doctor ever suggested it?" The truth is too few doctors talk to their patients about the importance of exercise despite the fact that the U.S. Preventive Services Task Force advises all doctors in primary care to discuss the benefits of exercise with their patients. Since doctors often cite lack of time or knowledge as the reason they don't follow through, we recommend instead that you talk to your doctor about exercise.

This is especially important if you are beginning an exercise program for the first time. Most people can begin to exercise moderately without a stress test (which measures heart function as you exercise on a treadmill). But it's wise to share your plans with your doctor, who knows you and your medical history. In some cases it's imperative to consult your doctor first: if you have a known medical condition such as heart disease or diabetes, or if you are a man over 40 or a woman over 50 who has done little or no exercise in the past.

SMART STUFF

Recently completed studies at the University of Wisconsin showed that when a person is active, the fat eaten in a meal tended to be burned for energy. In inactive people, the amount of fat burned was lower and it was more likely to be stored as body fat.

Ten Minutes at a Time

Can you spare 10 minutes? Most of us can. That's all it takes to get started. Rather than pushing people to get 30 minutes of exercise a day in one session, researchers recently discovered that the same benefits can be achieved from shorter sessions. Three 10-minute activity segments, broken up during the day, can achieve as much weight loss and almost as much in the way of health benefits as one 30-minute session. And those minutes add up to pounds lost quicker than you realize.

Fitting Fitness In

Activity	Minutes	Days/Week	Pounds/Year*
Walking	10	7	5
Bicycling	10	3	2
Gardening	10	2	2
Washing windows	10	1	1
Total Weight Loss			10

Lose 10 Pounds in a Year!

*Based on 150-pound person

WALK OFF WEIGHT

Walking is man's best medicine.

—Hippocrates

Most of us can walk—from the end of the parking lot, around the mall, through the building at work, around the neighborhood, or in the park—but we don't. The average American walks 1.4 miles a week—barely 1000 feet a day.

Walking

- Burns calories
- Builds muscles
- Builds bone
- Prevents colds
- Reduces the effects of aging
- Increases mental sharpness
- Lengthens your life

A quarter of all trips we make are under a mile, but 75% of those trips are made by car. Though this may be partially habit, it's not totally our fault. Our post-World War II vehicle-friendly suburbs often lack sidewalks, bike paths, parks, public transportation or shopping centers that we can reach on foot. Serious health problems and an epidemic of obesity may be an unanticipated by-product of the modern suburbs we've built. Study after study has shown that suburban residents walk less, bike less and are less physically fit than their city cousins. Many public health officials and community planners are currently working to redesign neighborhoods in order to encourage more outdoor activity.

Even without sidewalks, there are places we can walk: in shopping malls; through a large supermarket; around a museum, park or zoo; around and through the building at work; on the track at the local school; or on a treadmill. Walking is perfect exercise. It doesn't require any special talent or equipment, it can be done at any age and at a pace that's comfortable for you, and the risk of injury is almost nonexistent.

Start with a 10-minute walk. Begin by warming up for 2 to 3 minutes at a leisurely pace to help your heart rate adjust to the activity. Pick up the pace for 6 minutes and slow down for the last two. As you become more fit and add more time and distance, the beginning and end of each walk should remain the same with the middle getting longer and more vigorous.

Brisk walking, at 3 to 4 mph (miles per hour), is considered a moderate intensity activity. To judge if you have reached this level you should be able to walk two miles in 30 to 40 minutes. Even if you are slower, you will burn calories and increase your fitness if you walk most days of the week.

SMART STUFF

Walking on a treadmill is slightly different from walking on solid ground. There are no natural ups and downs or wind resistance. If you add an incline, as little as 1%, you'll come closer to the benefits of a "real life" walk.

The Power of Three

All out-of-shape people resemble one another—they have little muscle tone and limited stamina. Physically fit people do not look alike. Being fit is how our bodies change when subjected to specific mechanical demands. Runners look different from football players. And swimmers don't resemble wrestlers.

Fit people have many things in common. For everyone, getting fit produces positive changes in our cells, organs, muscles, blood and bones. In practical terms, fitness means you can climb stairs or carry heavy packages without becoming out of breath. The fitter you are, the less stress you put on your body when you are active.

The optimum road to fitness is a triad, or threesome, of activities recommended by the American College of Sports Medicine (ACSM): 1) aerobic exercise for cardiovascular conditioning,

2) strength training for muscle toning, and 3) flexibility to improve range of motion for your joints and muscles.

Aerobic exercises, or endurance activities. are those that increase your heart rate and breathing for an extended period of time. They include walking, swimming, bicycling, dancing, jogging or aerobic exercise classes like kick boxing, tai bo, and spinning. ACSM recommends a minimum of 20 minutes, 3 to 5 days a week. Intermittent bouts of ten minutes of exercise accumulated throughout the day is another way to reach the goal. The intensity of the exercise should be vigorous but not so intense that you are breathless and cannot talk. You should never be in pain or feel dizzy, light-headed, and nauseated.

SMART STUFF—How are you doing?
Write down how far you can walk in 10 minutes (in feet, blocks, laps, miles, or even the number of times you walk up and down a long hallway). Do this test again at the end of each month. As your endurance improves you should find you can walk farther in those 10 minutes.

Strength training, also called resistance training or weight training, are exercises that build muscle, improve strength, and stimulate the growth of bone. Even small changes in muscle size, an increase that is not visible, can make a big difference in strength. Most important, muscles are always active, so increasing them uses up calories, even when you are asleep.

Strength training can be accomplished in a number of ways. You can use special resistance machines (Cybex, Nautilus, Universal), free weights, resistance bands (giant bands you stretch to build muscle) or calisthenics (like sit-ups, leg lifts and push-ups). Some people enjoy combining them all for variety. ACSM recommends at least one set of 8 to 10 different exercises that condition the major muscle groups, done 2 to 3 days a week.

In Appendix 2, we've provided a basic strength training program with instructions to get you started. Your local "Y" or fitness center is another good resource as are instructional videos. Or you might consider treating yourself to a few sessions with a personal trainer.

SMART STUFF—Your trainer should be trained
Make sure the personal trainer you work with is certified by ACSM, the American Council on Exercise or the Aerobics and Fitness Association of America. Certified athletic trainers (ATC), exercise physiologists, physical educators, and physical therapists are other exercise professionals who are qualified to help you set up a personalized exercise program.

Flexibility, or stretching exercises, loosen muscles, allowing you full range of motion in all your joints. This helps you to perform any activity better, reduces the chance of injury and is a powerful weapon against aging. Yoga and tai chi are formal stretching programs but basic stretching exercises can be done anywhere—they make a great accompaniment to TV viewing. If you stretch to the point of mild pressure or discomfort, but not pain, holding each stretch 20 seconds, it is virtually impossible to hurt yourself.

ACSM recommends you stretch the major muscle groups 2 or 3 times a week. To get you started we've also provided a basic stretching program in Appendix 2.

It's Not True

- Weight gain is inevitable as you age.

    As we get older, as a result of inactivity, our percentage of body fat increases and the amount of muscle decreases, resulting in a decreased calorie need and an increase in body weight, but exercise fights both problems by burning calories and maintaining muscles. It is possible to gain weight as you age but not inevitable.

- No pain, no gain.

This is an outdated notion. Feeling a burn or pain when you exercise is not the best way to get results. All activity counts. Whether you jog for 20 minutes or walk for 40, you'll burn the same amount of calories. Slow or fast is not the issue, it's being active every day that counts in the long haul.

- Exercise can be dangerous, if you are older.

Researchers have developed successful strength training programs for nursing home residents proving it's never too late to get fit. The key is to start slow and proceed at your own pace.

- If you stop exercising, you'll lose all you've gained.

Research has proven that the benefits of exercise last longer than we ever imagined. If you stop exercising for a few weeks or even a month, you'll lose very little of your progress. Just take your workout down a notch from where you were when your took the hiatus and start again.

The Fidget Factor

Researchers have long pondered the question of why some people appear to gain weight easily while others, who eat the same amount, rarely put on pounds. One answer to the dilemma may be the "fidget factor"—finger tapping, leg jiggling, foot wiggling, or gum chewing. Those everyday habits burn calories, sometimes as many as a few hundred, on any given day. These activities are not typically measured by standard activity tests, but nonetheless they use up calories. Researchers have dubbed these spontaneous ordinary motions "non-exercise activity thermogenesis" or NEAT. If you are not already a fidgeter, it's unlikely you'll turn into one, but the next time you nervously tap your pencil on your desk, don't stop. It's NEAT and you're burning calories!

SMART STUFF—Even laughing counts!
Hearty laughing stimulates muscles throughout your body, increases the oxygen in your blood and increases your breathing rate. It's equal to light aerobic exercise.

Your Activity Goal

In Chapter 7, you'll set up your own personalized activity goal. Depending on whether you are currently inactive, somewhat active or moderately active, you'll be aiming to use up 500 to 1000 calories a week through activity and as you become more fit, your ultimate goal will be doubling this amount.

In Appendix 1, you'll find a Weekly Activity Log to record your daily activity and the chart Using Up Calories Through Activity to track the calories you've burned. Remember that activity has a two-fold benefit in your weight loss program: activity burns calories and activity builds muscles, which burn calories faster.

Tips to Keep You Motivated

- Join a group or club that includes activity: mall walkers, a walking or hiking group, tennis, golf, volleyball, softball, basketball, table tennis—the social aspect will keep you coming back.
- Design a screen saver that says: "Stop surfing, start sweating."
- Find a fitness buddy—walk together, golf together, join a gym. Activity loves company.
- Treat yourself to exercise equipment—free weights, a treadmill; they are frivolous if you don't use them but an investment if you do.
- Rent or borrow different exercise, yoga or stretching videos to add variety to your normal routine.
- Put exercise equipment in a spot where you pass it often throughout the day.
- Park your sneakers near the door as a reminder to walk instead of ride.
- Put a pad at the top and bottom of the stairs and make a check mark for every trip and the 10 calories you burn each time.
- Reward yourself for a job well done. One of our clients treated herself to a facial every time she exercised daily for two weeks and she said she had "Great skin to go along with a great bod." Another bought an expensive golf club.

- Expect setbacks: there are going to be times when you don't stick to your exercise program. That's normal; just get moving again as soon as you can.

Reinforce the Value of Exercise

- The simplest exercise program—**just move**.
- Walk whenever and wherever possible.
- For total fitness combine: aerobic exercise (to build endurance and stamina); strength training (to build muscles, gain strength and burn more calories); and flexibility (to increase range of motion).
- Fidget—every activity burns calories!
- Add activity to your day-to-day routine to achieve your activity goal.

Summing It Up

We know there is a lot of information to absorb in this chapter, but you will come back to it again and again to reinforce the secrets to successful weight loss. We always tell our clients that it takes effort to change habits and lose weight. But the effort will pay off. Some weight loss programs promise "no work" and insist the pounds will still melt away. That's just not true.

Get Skinny works. You'll use your three secrets to success—thin habits, commonsense portions and exercise—combined with proven natural dieting aids. You'll do this meal-by-meal, week-by-week and before you know it you'll be at your target weight.

SMART STUFF—Buddy-up

Studies have demonstrated that healthy living loves company. A buddy or a group of buddies offers encouragement, empathy and accountability. It's harder to make excuses or avoid regular exercise when someone else is counting on you for company and support. Your resolve to eat well is stronger when you have to share your latest meal choices with a buddy. Getting morale-boosting e-mails actually helped a group of university employees in a weight loss program make positive behavior changes and lose more weight than a control group.

Chapter 7

A Closer Look at You

Overweight is the second leading cause (after smoking)
of preventable death in the United States today.

—National Institutes of Health

Many diets give you a one-size-fits-all eating plan. We believe
that's why all of them work in the short term but fail in the long
run. You are not like everyone else. If everyone could be successful on the same eating plan, everyone would be slim. But the sad
fact is that over 55% of American adults are overweight.

So, before you start working toward being thinner, we want
you to take *a closer look at you!* What are your goals? What is your
weight history? What is your health history? How active are you?
What do you usually eat?

In this chapter you will take that closer look at yourself by
answering the questions on the following pages. Your answers
will ensure that you will win the losing game once and for all
because you will finally have an individualized eating plan tailored
to your needs and goals. By the end of this chapter you'll have
answers to the three questions that are the key to lifelong successful eating:

How am I doing—right now?

Where should I be headed?

How do I get there?

Over and over, throughout a lifetime of healthy eating, you can use the tools provided to assess where you are and where you need to go. At different times and in different circumstances the answers may change. But you're in charge. You ask the three essential questions. You get the answers.

How am I doing—right now?

Where should I be headed?

How do I get there?

And you set up an eating plan that is right for you and only you. We guarantee this approach will work every time. So, let's get started finding out all about you!

Mirror, Mirror, on the Wall

When was the last time you took a really good look at yourself, not just admiring a new outfit but actually looking at your body? It is important to have an accurate body image so that you can assess what you need to do to achieve your weight loss goals. The simplest way to do this is to remove all your clothes and stand in front of a full-length mirror.

What do you see? Do you recognize the person in the mirror? What do you like? What would you like to change? Don't squeeze your eyes shut and run from the room. You need to judge yourself carefully. All of us have figure faults, places where fat deposits or places where we are too lean. One of our clients once moaned, "My mom was so lucky. When she was my age hips were in style."

Style often plays a part in what we expect from ourselves. If the current style is an angular or straight look, it can be discouraging if you have a more curvy body type. Take a close look at you. If you have more rolls and pouches than you had in the past, it's time to take control. No one can guarantee you a movie star figure, but we can guarantee you a slimmer, healthier body.

While you are using *Get Skinny*'s eating and exercise plan, go back to the mirror every few weeks or so. You'll be pleasantly surprised at the changes you see.

Always on a Diet?

For as long as you can remember, you've been on a diet. Does that statement apply to you? Well, you're not alone. It is estimated that on any given day over half the adults in America are dieting. Just listen to any group of people talking and you're bound to hear someone giving dieting advice or a testimony about a miraculous weight loss plan that someone just started. If everyone is dieting, why are we getting heavier and heavier with each passing year? Perhaps it's because everyone is using a one-size-fits-all diet plan instead of setting up a program that is meant for them and them alone. But that is about to change with *Your Personalized Weight Attack Plan,* which is tailored to fit your needs. You begin by looking at your weight history. You need to know where you've been before you know where you need to go.

Your Weight History

1. ____ At what age did you begin to weigh more than you should for your size?

____ How old are you now?

____ How many years have you weighed too much?

2. Do you diet

____ All the time

____ Most of the time

____ To lose weight only for a special occasion

____ Rarely if ever

3. When you diet, which type of diet would you most likely follow?

____ Fasting

____ Eating no fat or lowfat foods

____ Cutting out or limiting certain types of foods

____ Drastically cutting down portion sizes of all foods

____ Skipping meals

4. After you diet and you go back to your regular eating pattern do you

____ Gain back the weight you lost, plus some extra

____ Gain back the weight you lost

____ Maintain your weight loss

Maintaining a sensible weight is tough. Three or more times a day you have to face *food*. It would be so easy if you could simply stop eating. One of our clients once told us he envied alcoholics because they could control their problem by staying away from alcohol for the rest of their life. He couldn't stop eating.

That attitude can be part of the problem. Many overweight people see food as an enemy, not an ally. *Get Skinny* will help you turn a former enemy into your strongest support. Not food itself but how much and how often you eat can be the reason you've never been able to win the "weight war." All that is about to change. *Get Skinny* will never ask you to fast for a day, skip meals or give up any foods. In fact, on the *Get Skinny* diet *no foods are forbidden*.

Your Best BMI

Body mass index, or BMI, is used to estimate health risk; it has been used for years as a research tool. As your BMI goes up so does your risk for early death and serious illness including: heart disease, high blood pressure, stroke, diabetes, gallbladder disease, arthritis, sleep apnea, and breast and endometrial cancer.

Guidelines revised in 1998, by the National Heart, Lung and Blood Institute (NHLBI) of the National Institutes of Health (NIH), recommend that adults aim for a BMI below 25. A BMI of 18.5 to 24.9 is considered normal. A BMI of less than 18.5 is considered underweight. Those with BMIs between 25 and 30 are considered overweight, while those with BMIs over 30 are classified as significantly overweight. It's estimated that 55 percent of adults have BMIs in the 25 and over range. According to these guidelines a staggering 97 million Americans weigh too much!

BMI is a better way to measure the amount of body fat than traditional height–weight tables. For a person 5 feet, 4 inches tall, a BMI of 24 equals 140 pounds; a BMI of 30 equals 175 pounds. For a person 5 feet, 10 inches, a BMI of 24 equals 175 pounds; a BMI of 30 equals 205 pounds. Body mass index is calculated by dividing your body weight in kilograms by height in meters squared or you can simply use the following chart.

YOUR BODY MASS INDEX (BMI)

Experts recommend a BMI below 25.

Find your height on the left of the chart. Find the weight nearest your weight across the top of the chart. Follow the weight column down and the height column across until they meet. Your BMI is the number at the intersection of your weight and height.

Your BMI is _____

Weight	100	105	110	115	120	125	130	135	140	145	150	155	160	165	170	175	180	185	190	195	200	205
Height																						
5'0"	20	21	21	22	23	24	**25**	26	27	28	29	30	31	32	33	34	35	36	37	38	39	40
5'1"	19	20	21	22	23	24	**25**	26	26	27	28	29	30	31	32	33	34	35	36	37	38	39
5'2"	18	19	20	21	22	23	24	**25**	26	27	27	28	29	30	31	32	33	34	35	36	37	37
5'3"	18	19	19	20	21	22	23	24	**25**	26	27	27	28	29	30	31	32	33	34	35	35	36
5'4"	17	18	19	20	21	21	22	23	24	**25**	26	27	27	28	29	30	31	32	33	33	34	35
5'5"	17	17	18	19	20	21	22	22	23	24	**25**	26	27	27	28	29	30	31	32	32	33	34
5'6"	16	17	18	19	19	20	21	22	23	23	24	**25**	26	27	27	28	29	30	31	31	32	33
5'7"	16	16	17	18	19	20	20	21	22	23	23	24	**25**	26	27	27	28	29	30	31	31	32
5'8"	15	16	17	17	18	19	20	21	21	22	23	24	24	**25**	26	27	27	28	29	30	30	31
5'9"	15	16	16	17	18	18	19	20	21	21	22	23	24	24	**25**	26	27	27	28	29	30	30
5'10"	14	15	16	17	17	18	19	19	20	21	22	22	23	24	24	**25**	26	27	27	28	29	30
5'11"	14	15	15	16	17	17	18	19	20	20	21	22	22	23	24	24	**25**	26	26	27	28	29
6'0"	14	14	15	16	16	17	18	18	19	20	20	21	22	22	23	24	24	**25**	26	26	27	28
6'1"	13	14	15	15	16	16	17	18	18	19	20	20	21	22	22	23	24	24	**25**	26	26	27
6'2"	13	13	14	15	15	16	17	17	18	19	19	20	21	21	22	22	23	24	24	**25**	26	26
6'3"	12	13	14	14	15	16	16	17	17	18	19	19	20	21	21	22	22	23	24	24	**25**	26
6'4"	12	13	13	14	15	15	16	16	17	18	18	19	19	20	21	21	22	23	23	24	24	**25**

BMI is not a foolproof way to measure overweight. A person with a very muscular, dense body build and a low percentage of body fat could end up with the same BMI as someone who truly is overweight, and who has a high percentage of body fat. One way to sort out the difference is to measure waistlines. The NIH guidelines say that those with a BMI of 25 to 35, and with waistlines of 40 inches or more for men and 35 inches or more for women, face increased health risks. Fat that collects around the belly should be considered a serious health threat.

Rate Your Health Risks

There is an old saying, "You can pick your friends but not your relatives." What does this have to do with dieting, you ask? Well, those relatives contributed to your gene package and your genes will dictate, to some degree, the health risks you face and the health benefits you enjoy. It is important to have a complete picture of your health history.

Your Health Risks Quiz

Circle the answer that best applies to you. You may not know the answers to every question. That's fine, just skip the ones you don't know and go on. (For scoring purposes not every question has three answer options.)

Family History

1. One or more close blood relatives (parents, grandparents, siblings) is overweight.
   A. No family members are overweight.
   B. Few family members are overweight.
   C. Numerous family members are overweight.

2. One or more close blood relatives has had a heart attack or stroke.
   A. No family history of heart attack or stroke
   B. After age 55
   C. Before age 55

3. One or more close blood relatives has had diabetes.
   A. No family history of diabetes
   B. After age 60
   C. Before age 60

4. One or more close blood relatives has had cancer.
   A. No family history of cancer
   B. After age 75
   C. Before age 75

5. One or more close blood relatives has experienced signs of osteoporosis.
   A. No family history of osteoporosis
   B. Lost height
   C. Lost height and fractured a bone

Personal History

6. Have you ever had a heart attack or stroke?
   A. No
   C. Yes

7. Do you have diabetes?
   A. No
   C. Yes

8. Have you had cancer?
   A. No
   C. Yes

9. Have you been overweight?
   A. Only for the last 3–5 years
   B. Most of your adult life
   C. Most of your life

10. Your current weight is
    A. Less than 5 pounds from your target weight
    B. 5 to 14 pounds over your target weight
    C. 15 or more pounds over your target weight

11. Your current BMI (body mass index) is
    A. Less than 25
    B. 25 to 30
    C. Over 30

12. Your total cholesterol level is
    A. Below 200 mg/dl
    B. 200 to 239 mg/dl
    C. 240 mg/dl or higher

13. Your LDL (low-density lipoprotein) level is
    A. Below 130 mg/dl
    B. 130 to 159 mg/dl
    C. 160 mg/dl or higher

14. Your blood pressure is
    A. Lower than 130/85
    B. Between 130/85 and 159/99
    C. Higher than 160/100

15. You smoke
    A. Never smoked or quit more than ten years ago
    B. Less than one pack a day or you quit one to 10 years ago
    C. One or more packs a day

16. You exercise
    A. 30 minutes three or more times a week
    B. 30 minutes once or twice a week
    C. Occasionally or not at all

17. Stress
    A. You are easygoing and seldom rushed or irritable
    B. You are sometimes impatient, rushed or irritable
    C. You are easily angered, often mistrustful, impatient or irritable

18. You practice other good health habits, like flossing your teeth, using sun screen, and wearing seat belts.
    A. All the time
    B. Most of the time
    C. Rarely or never

Rate Your Health Risks

Add up the number of As, Bs and Cs you circled and write them below.

A answers _____   B answers _____   C answers _____

"A" answers signal the least risk. "B" answers signal moderate risk. And "C" answers indicate the most risk . If more than a third (6 out of 18) of your answers are Cs, it's time to make some positive changes in your life to reduce your health risks. If more than half (9 out of 18) of your answers are Bs, you have some health risks that you can minimize and you will definitely benefit from using *Get Skinny.*

While you can't change your family history, by adjusting your eating behavior and lifestyle habits, you can reduce and even prevent some of the health consequences that have troubled other family members. Every positive effort you make to eat well and live well will pay off in health benefits.

Let's take a closer look at the risks you noted in questions 6 through 18.

6, 7, 8, 9, 10, 11—*Maintaining your target weight is one of the most important things you can do to minimize your risk of illness.* It's simple—extra pounds = added risk for heart disease, diabetes and cancer. Losing weight, even as little as five pounds (which may be far less than your target), will help to reduce your risk for these serious health problems.

12—High blood cholesterol levels have been identified as an important risk factor for heart disease. In recent years, Americans have become more aware of the importance of cholesterol and the average adult blood cholesterol level has come down. But still, one in five adults has a cholesterol level that is too high. Losing weight and lowering the total amount of fat you eat are the two best ways to lower your total cholesterol.

13—Today, your doctor will look not only at your total cholesterol number but at the proportion of HDLs (high density lipoproteins) and LDLs (low density lipoproteins) that make up the total number. LDL cholesterol is often referred to as "bad" cholesterol because it's the type that frequently gets deposited in the artery walls. Higher levels of LDLs are associated with an increased risk of heart disease. Losing weight, exercising regularly and not smoking are among the best things you can do to lower your LDLs.

14—Blood pressure is the force of blood against the artery walls. It is reported as two numbers written like this: 120/80. The first figure (systolic pressure) is the maximum pressure when the heart contracts. The second number (diastolic pressure) is the minimum pressure when the heart relaxes between beats. The higher your blood pressure, the greater your risk for heart disease. Overweight people are more likely to have high blood pressure. Losing as little as five pounds can have a dramatic effect on your blood pressure. Don't smoke and add regular exercise and the results will be even greater.

15—There is nothing positive to say about smoking. Smokers age quicker and die younger. Smoking even lessens your enjoyment of food by blunting your sense of taste. If you smoke, do yourself a favor and stop.

16—*Get Skinny* stresses exercise as a prime weapon in the battle of the bulge. If you exercise regularly, not only will you be slimmer, you'll have a more positive attitude toward life and you'll be less likely to suffer from serious illness.

17—The role stress plays in your overall health is controversial. Research has shown that external stresses do not harm you as much as being angry, hostile or mistrustful. Irritability significantly increases a person's risk for heart disease. As a reaction to stress, some people eat to calm down. As we examine health from a more holistic view, it is obvious that stress has a negative impact on quality of life, so efforts to reduce stress are important. Regular exercise is a great way to blow off steam.

18—People who regularly practice simple, good health habits like flossing their teeth, using sunscreen and wearing seat belts, often carry these good behaviors over into other aspects of their lives, like exercising regularly and eating well. Every positive effort you make will pay off in health benefits.

Rate Your Activity

We are a country of people who exert as little energy as possible. We drive to work, take the elevator to our floor, send e-mails to office mates, and send out for lunch. At home, machines wash our clothes and dishes, open cans, mix food, answer the telephone, and change channels. And the future promises even more labor-saving devices. Though the conveniences are great, they come at an enormous cost. We are a country of out-of-shape, overweight people. Most of us spend more time in our seat than on our feet.

Rate Your Activity Level

Circle the answer that best applies to you.

1. The type of physical activity involved in my job or daily routine is best described by the following:

A. My typical day involves at least 1 hour of vigorous physical activity (running, bicycling, rollerblading, hammering or chopping wood).

B. My typical day involves at least 30 minutes of moderate physical activity (walking, swimming, aerobic exercise class, vacuuming, gardening).

C. My typical day involves office work or light household chores (filing, typing, dusting, folding laundry).

2. I participate in at least 30 minutes of activity (walking, running, swimming, dancing, exercise classes, bicycling, rollerblading, basketball)

A. Five to seven times a week

B. Two or three times a week

C. Rarely or never

3. I participate in yoga, tai chi, or stretching exercises

A. At least 2 times a week

B. One or less times a week

C. Rarely or never

4. I participate in strength training exercises (free weights or resistance machines)

A. At least 2 to 3 times a week

B. One or less times a week

C. Rarely or never

5. I enjoy recreational sports activities (golf, tennis, volleyball, dancing, table tennis)

A. Once or twice a week

B. Once or twice a month

C. Never

6. When I feel stressed, I use exercise to relax

A. Often

B. Occasionally

C. Never

Rate Your Activity

Add up the number of As, Bs and Cs you circled and write them below.

A answers _____   B answers _____   C answers _____

Your "A" answers show that you exercise regularly. Check below to see if you are on target for the FITT formula. "B" answers signal a moderate interest in exercise with no real exercise plan in place. It is time to get serious about this part of your health plan. The reward you'll reap from regular exercise is that the pounds will come off quicker and stay off easier. "C" answers indicate that it's time for you to get moving! Lack of regular activity contributes to extra weight and poor health. As we said in Chapter 6, muscles use more calories than fat. Exercising sheds fat while building muscle and the end result is that your body burns more calories. You feel better, look better and use calories faster.

In Chapter 6 there is much more information about exercise and it's importance to your overall health and weight loss goals. A nice starting point, to get you going right now, is the FITT formula.

F = Frequency

Start by planning some physical activity three times a week and add more days slowly until you are active every day of the week.

I = Intensity

Intensity is a measure of how hard you exercise. Go at a pace that is right for you. It is more important to move slowly, at first, than not move at all. Bill Bowerman, the inventor of Nike shoes and a famous track coach at the University of Oregon, recommends that you talk while you exercise. If you can't hold a conversation, the pace is too fast for you.

T = Time

Start by trying to be active continuously for 10 minutes. Gradually, you can extend the length of your activity until you reach 30 minutes. Research has shown that you do not need to get 30 minutes of continuous activity to receive a benefit. The 30 minutes can be cumulative in amounts of less time. The key is to build movement into your day.

T = Type

You won't move if you don't enjoy it. The choices of activities are endless. You need to find something that you enjoy and that gives you a sense of well-being and satisfaction. And remember, variety is the spice of life—vary your activity so you stay interested.

Rate What's on Your Plate

If fibbing about what we eat burned calories, Americans would be a thin bunch. In a survey by Wirthlin Worldwide, people were asked to compare their current diet to what they ate two or three years ago. Of the adults surveyed, 55% reported eating lowfat foods more often, 61% said they eat more high-fiber foods, 76% claimed to be eating more fruits and vegetables, 49% said they are eating less red meat, 67% report cutting back on fast foods, and 59% said they indulge in snacks and treats less often. These self-reported answers do not jibe with USDA food consumption studies that show: American adults are not as interested in eating lowfat foods as they once were; the average fiber intake is half what it should be; and French fries are still America's "favorite" vegetable. Steak restaurants are enjoying a resurgence of popularity and it's estimated that 76% of Americans snack daily.

If you are serious about losing weight, and we know you are, then it is important to accurately examine what's on your plate.

How Does Your Plate Rate?

Circle the answer that best applies to you.

1. I eat three meals a day
   A. Every day
   B. Most days
   C. Rarely

2. I eat breakfast
   A. Always
   B. Most days
   C. Rarely

3. I'm interested in trying new foods
   A. Always
   B. Usually
   C. Rarely

4. I try to make good snack choices (such as fruit, yogurt, pretzels)
   A. Always
   B. Most of the time
   C. Rarely

5. I try to drink enough water each day
   A. 8 to 10 cups
   B. Less than 8 cups
   C. I drink very little water daily

6. I eat pies, cakes, cookies, doughnuts, candy
   A. Occasionally
   B. 2 to 3 times a week
   C. Almost every day

7. I eat chips, peanuts, buttered popcorn, snack mix, snack crackers
   A. Occasionally
   B. 2 to 3 times a week
   C. Almost every day

8. I eat fried foods
   A. Occasionally
   B. 2 to 3 times a week
   C. More than 3 times a week

9. I choose reduced fat varieties of margarine, mayonnaise, sour cream, cream and salad dressing
   A. Almost always
   B. Occasionally
   C. Rarely if ever

10. I almost always choose
    A. Nonfat (skim) milk
    B. 1% or 2% fat milk
    C. Whole milk

11. I almost always choose:
    A. Reduced fat cheese
    B. Some reduced fat and some regular cheese
    C. Regular full fat cheese

12. I almost always choose
    A. Nonfat ice cream, nonfat frozen yogurt, sherbet, and sorbet
    B. Reduced fat ice cream and frozen yogurt
    C. Premium (full-fat) ice cream

13. I eat grain-based foods (bread, cereal, rice, pasta)
    A. 5 to 7 servings a day
    B. Less than 5 servings a day
    C. I rarely eat this group of foods

14. I eat whole grain breads, cereal, rice, pasta
    A. Most of the time
    B. Occasionally
    C. Rarely

15. I eat 2 to 3 servings of vegetables (broccoli, salad, tomatoes, carrots, zucchini) each day
    A. Always
    B. Most of the time
    C. Rarely

16. I eat 2 to 3 servings of fruit (apple, mango, grapefruit, grapes) and fruit juice each day
    A. Always
    B. Most of the time
    C. Rarely

17. I eat at least one excellent source of vitamin C (orange, grapefruit, tomato, or their juices, strawberries, cantaloupe, broccoli, green peppers) each day

A. Always
B. Most of the time
C. Rarely

18. I eat at least two excellent sources of calcium each day (milk, yogurt, cheese, calcium-fortified soy milk, calcium-fortified juice)
   A. Always
   B. Most of the time
   C. Rarely

19. I select lean protein choices (extra lean chopped meat, chicken without skin, fish, shellfish, pork loin, flank and round steak)
   A. Always
   B. Most of the time
   C. Rarely

20. I eat beans
   A. Often
   B. Occasionally
   C. Rarely

21. I eat hot dogs, sausage, bacon, salami, bologna
   A. Once in a while
   B. Once or twice a week
   C. Five or more times a week

22. I limit beer, wine and liquor to no more than 1 drink a day for women and 2 drinks a day for men
   A. Always
   B. Usually
   C. I regularly have more than 1 drink a day

23. I eat when I'm hungry, not when the clock says it's mealtime
   A. Always
   B. Most of the time
   C. I rarely feel hungry

24. I eat late in the evening or in the middle of the night
   A. Rarely if ever
   B. Once in a while
   C. Regularly

25. When I'm upset
    A. I try to find nonfood options to channel my emotions
    B. I sometimes find comfort in food
    C. I often find comfort in food

Rate Your Plate

Add up the number of As, Bs and Cs you circled and write them below.

A answers _____   B answers _____   C answers _____

"A" answers signal you make good food choices almost all the time. Keep up the good work. "B" answers signal that you are heading in the right direction but you need to be more conscious of your food choices. And "C" answers indicate that you give little thought to what you eat. If more than a third (9 out of 25) of your answers are Cs, it's time to make some positive changes in what you eat so you reduce your weight and health risks. If more than half (13 out of 25) of your answers are Bs, you have already begun to eat better but you can do even more to achieve your goal of losing weight and being healthier. Following the *Get Skinny* diet guarantees you'll achieve the goals you've set.

The wonderful thing about rating what's on your plate is that you are in total control. What you eat, when you eat, and how much you eat are behavior patterns that you can change and adapt so that eating becomes your best ally. You may have already noticed that no question on the quiz How Does Your Plate Rate? suggested that you should give up a food or category of foods. That's because, as we've said before on the *Get Skinny* diet, "no foods are forbidden"—ever!

Every positive effort you make to eat better will pay off in positive results. You'll watch your weight go down and your energy go up.

1—Our bodies are like machines that need care, attention and a source of energy. Eating at regular intervals throughout the day helps your body work at peak performance while discouraging you from the "feast and famine" routine—skipping some meals only to overload at others.

2—Did you know that breakfast eaters are leaner, have lower blood pressures, get a wider variety of nutrients throughout the day, have less midmorning fatigue, and may even think better than non-breakfast eaters? That's a pretty good endorsement for an A.M. meal.

3—Adventurous eaters not only have a lot of fun trying new things but they add nutrients, fiber and taste to their meals. Adam Drewnowski, Ph.D., at the University of Washington in Seattle says that, ideally, we should be eating 8 different foods each day. His research has shown that many women eat only 6 to 10 different foods over a two week span of time. People tend to eat the same small group of foods over and over again.

4—There is nothing wrong with snacking. Regular snackers are often leaner than nonsnackers because they are more likely to eat when they are hungry rather than when habit or the clock says it's mealtime. The key is to select snacks that offer a nutrient bonus and are not packed with calories.

5—As you know from Chapter 5, water is one of your secret weapons in winning the diet game. Most experts recommend up to 8 glasses a day. Thirst and hunger are often confused, so when you feel like eating, a simple trick is to have a tall glass of water first and you'll be pleasantly surprised to find out how often you are satisfied.

6, 7, 8—All these foods, bite for bite, pack in more calories than healthier choices and they're loaded with salt, fat, or sugar. On *Get Skinny* we'll never tell you that you cannot eat these foods. We'll suggest instead that you put them in the "blue moon category." You can eat them once-in-a-blue-moon—occasionally.

9, 10, 11, 12—Full-fat versions contain the same nutrients but more calories and fat than the reduced fat or nonfat varieties. Bite for bite, foods high in fat can have over two times the calories of the nonfat version. By selecting lowfat or nonfat milk, cheese, ice cream, and salad dressing you save thousands of calories a year. If you switch from cream to skim milk in your coffee, it's been estimated that you eat 10,000 calories less in a year—the equivalent of almost three pounds of body weight!

13, 14, 15, 16, 17—Every food listed is rich in carbohydrates, vitamins and minerals and many offer fiber and antioxidants (natural body protectors) as well. Too often diets eliminate carbohydrates, shortchanging you of a valuable, quickly utilized source of energy, and many vital nutrients that offer protection against serious illness.

18—Calcium not only protects bones but is also vital to the functioning of your nerves and heart. Research has demonstrated that ample calcium helps you lose weight, may protect you against certain cancers, and is necessary in controlling blood pressure.

19, 20, 21—There is no question that protein is important—it tastes good and makes you feel full longer. The key is not to eat huge portions, which could crowd out other important foods in a meal. Try eating plant-based protein sources more often and save high fat protein sources for once-in-a-blue-moon.

22—The role of alcohol in health is controversial but the evidence is mounting that a small amount—about 1 drink a day—is beneficial.

23, 24, 25—Eating is a complex behavior and emotions can play a big role. A study from Yale University found that women who had more trouble dealing with stressful situations had more fat around their middle. If your emotions regularly interplay with the way you eat, you need to identify this and adapt your behavior. Every positive change you make will pay off in lost weight.

Your Starting Line for *Your Personalized Weight Attack Plan*

"How Am I Doing—Right Now?"

Your Health Risks

Record the number of A, B and C answers from Your Health Risks quiz on page 108.

A answers _____   B answers _____   C answers _____

Check all that apply.

I need to: ____ Lose weight

____ Lose weight and lower my BMI

____ Make eating and lifestyle changes to lower my total cholesterol

____ Make eating and lifestyle changes to lower LDL cholesterol

____ Make eating and lifestyle changes to lower my blood pressure

____ Stop smoking

____ Begin exercising

____ Exercise on a regular basis

____ Practice stress reduction techniques

____ Practice simple good health habits like wearing seat belts

Your Goal: To modify your lifestyle and eating behaviors to change your "C" answers to "As" and "Bs."

Every few weeks, rate your risks again to evaluate how you've progressed. The ultimate goal is to have all "A" answers. Don't expect to change overnight. But remember, every positive change you make will have a positive impact on your health.

Your BMI

Your BMI is ____ (see page 104).
Your Goal: To modify your lifestyle and eating behavior to lower your BMI below 25.

Rate Your Activity

Record the number of A, B and C answers from the Rate Your Activity Level quiz on page 112.

A answers _____   B answers _____   C answers _____

Check all that apply.

I need to: ____ Exercise daily

____ Get involved in some type of stretching activity

____ Set up a strength training program

____ Get involved in some type of recreational sports

____ Use exercise as a stress reducer

If you answered "A" to question 1—"My typical day involves at least 1 hour of vigorous physical activity."—you are either an extremely active person or you have a very physically active job. That's great because you more than exceed the daily recommendations for activity. You may want to consider your level of aerobic, continuous activity, such as walking or bicycling, and your level of flexibility.

Every few weeks, rate your activity level again to see how you have progressed. The ultimate goal is to have all "A" answers. Don't expect yourself to change overnight. But remember, every positive change you make will have a positive impact on your weight, health and level of stress.

Your Goal: To incorporate exercise into your daily life so that all your answers to questions 2 through 6 are "As."

Rate What's on Your Plate

Record the number of A, B and C answers from the Rate What's on Your Plate quiz on page 117.

A answers _____   B answers _____   C answers _____

Check all that apply.

I need to: ____ Eat regular meals every day

____ Eat breakfast every day

____ Add more variety to my food choices

____ Make better snack choices

____ Drink more water every day

____ Cut down on fried food choices

____ Use more reduced fat or nonfat food choices

____ Eat more grain-based foods

____ Eat more vegetables

____ Eat more fruits

____ Eat more calcium-rich foods

____ Eat lean and plant-based protein foods

____ Identify my emotional response to eating

Your Goal: To modify your eating behavior to change your "C" answers to "As" and "Bs."

Every few weeks, rate your plate again to evaluate how you've progressed. The ultimate goal is to have all "A" answers. Don't expect to change overnight. But remember, every positive eating change you make will have a positive impact on your weight and health.

"Where Should I Be Headed?"

Finding Your Target Weight

You probably already have a pretty good idea of what you'd like to weigh and how much you need to lose to get there—5 pounds,

15 pounds, maybe even 30 or more. When you can't comfortably wear most of the clothes in your closet you know it's time to get serious about losing weight.

There are a number of ways to find your target weight. You already know there are health advantages to having a BMI below 25. Your target weight can simply be the weight for your height that corresponds with a BMI of 24. (See Your Body Mass Index, page 104.)

How much did you weigh in your early twenties? If you were a normal weight then, that's probably a good weight to maintain throughout your adult life. Few of us are as trim and slim as we were at twenty-five. The changing demands of our busy lives seem to have a way of showing up around our hips and stomachs. Most of us would love to weigh what we did in our twenties and for most of us that is an achievable goal. If so, then your target weight can be what you weighed in your early twenties.

Another way to "guesstimate" your target weight is an easy-to-use formula based on your height.

For Women: Give yourself 100 pounds for the first 5 feet of your height and add 5 pounds for each additional inch (or subtract 5 pounds for each inch under 5 feet). For example, if you're 5 feet, 4 inches tall:

100 pounds (for the first 5 feet of height)
* 20 pounds (5 pounds for every inch over 5 feet; 5 × 4 = 20)*
——
120 pounds is a desirable target weight

For Men: Give yourself 106 pounds for the first 5 feet of your height and add 6 pounds for each additional inch over 5 feet. For example, if you're 5 feet, 10 inches tall:

106 pounds (for the first 5 feet of height)
* 60 pounds (6 pounds for every inch over 5 feet; 6 × 10 = 60)*
——
166 pounds is a desirable target weight

Your Target Weight

Your target weight is: _____
Your goal: To modify your eating and activity behavior to achieve your target weight. Be patient with yourself. Change is hard but we guarantee that if you stick with *Your Personalized Weight Attack Plan,* you'll reach your target.

Target Your Calorie Zone

Calories are calories, no matter where they come from—apples or chocolate fudge. Every time you eat, you get calories. It doesn't matter if the food is high in carbohydrate, protein or fat. All foods have calories. (Water and most fibers are the exceptions.) While it is true that fat is a more concentrated source of calories than carbohydrate and protein, most foods are combinations, so when you eat a meal or snack you often get all three.

Studies have shown, over and over, that if you cut calories you lose weight. It doesn't matter if those calories are from protein, fat or carbohydrate. When you take in more calories than you need, you gain weight.

That's why it is so important for you to **target your calorie zone**—the number of calories you need to eat each day to reach your target weight.

Targeting Your Calorie Zone

1. Select your calorie factor:
   Select the factor that best suits you:
   - 20 = Very active men
   - 15 = Moderately active men or very active women
   - 13 = Inactive men, moderately active women and all people over age 55
   - 10 = Inactive women, repeat dieters, seriously overweight people

2. Find your target calorie zone:
Target weight x calorie factor = Target calorie zone
130 (target weight) × 13 (moderately active woman) =
1690 calories a day

For example, if your target weight is 130 and you are a moderately active woman, your target calorie zone would be 1600 to 1700 calories a day. Eating this amount of calories each day would guarantee weight loss. Couple this with daily activity and the weight comes off even faster.

Calories count! Any diet plan that tells you otherwise is not being truthful and is not based in scientific research on how the body works. Your body needs energy to function and to repair the wear and tear of daily living. This energy is received through calories, which are derived from the foods you eat.

Eat the right amount of calories and your body uses them to keep humming along. There are no extras to store and no deficit to make up. Eat too many calories and your body uses what it needs and stores the remaining energy for future use. A good deal of this storage is obvious on your thighs, hips and waist. Eat too few calories and your body draws on its energy stores to meet demands. Suddenly, your thighs, hips and waist get smaller as your energy surplus is depleted.

SMART STUFF—Do you burn calories thinking?
Using your brain does require energy but in such small amounts that unfortunately, it plays little or no role in weight loss. Experts at the Harvard Medical School, Department of Psychiatry suggest the role the brain does play in weight loss is to provide the state of mind and motivation needed to start a diet and exercise plan.

It can be hard to estimate calories because many foods you eat are combinations or you have no idea how they are prepared or you have trouble estimating the portion size. Even with these problems, it is important to have a rough idea of how many calories you are getting when you decide to eat a certain food.

In Chapter 6, you found out how to estimate serving sizes accurately. You know the difference between a portion (what you are served) and a serving (a standard measurement). You know that a portion of spaghetti might have as many as 2 to 3 servings. Understanding this distinction is vital to not overeating and not underestimating what you eat. You also found out in Chapter 6 that standard portions of many foods can be assigned caloric values that are fairly accurate. If you know how big a serving is and you know the approximate number of calories in a serving, you can estimate the number of calories you are eating.

In Chapter 8 you'll take A Closer Look at Food. This chapter is stuffed with hints, tips and tricks to help you select and prepare the healthiest foods. You know your calorie zone, you know how to estimate serving sizes and calories in an average serving, and soon you'll be an expert at selecting foods. As you put your new skills to work, you'll see the pounds fall away as your target weight gets closer and closer.

Your Target Calorie Zone

Your Target Weight ___ × Your Calorie Factor ___ =
  Your Target Calorie Zone

Your Target Calorie Zone is: ___

Your goal: To modify your eating behavior so that you consume approximately your target calorie zone daily. Add activity each day and you will use up even more of your energy stores (extra weight) so that you'll reach your target weight more quickly.

"How Do I Get There?"

Setting Your Weight Loss Goal

This is simple. If you currently weigh 153 pounds and your target weight is 130, you weight loss goal is 23 pounds.

Your weight loss goal

____ Current Weight
____ Target Weight

_____
____ Your Weight Loss Goal

Setting Your Activity Goals

Activity burns calories. For a person who is inactive, using up as little as 500 calories a week through activity can have health benefits. If you are a true couch potato, you need to start slowly, and this may be the level at which to start. Real health benefits start to click in when your use up 1,000 calories a week in moderate exercise. Consider 2,000 calories as a great goal to strive for over time.

Sounds great, you say, but how are you supposed to find all this extra time to exercise? First, start moving when you do have leisure time: instead of sitting through a movie, go ice skating; instead of going out for dinner, plan a hike and a picnic. And the really good news is that a study at Stanford University's School of Medicine showed that you can benefit from exercise whether the activity is continuous or done in bouts of activity. Brief activity, for as little as 10 minutes at a time, not only burns calories but also has a positive impact on your health—walking from the edge of the parking lot, climbing stairs instead of taking the escalator, washing windows and mowing the lawn all add to your daily activity total. The key is to *move* every day in some way.

Your activity goal

You are:
____ Inactive
____ Somewhat active
____ Moderately active

Inactive individuals should start by planning activities that burn at least 500 calories each week. After a few weeks, start increasing your activity goal to gradually reach 1000 calories each week.

Somewhat active individuals should begin by planning activities to use up at least 750 calories a week, gradually increasing that goal to 1500.

If you already exercise regularly, keep track of your activities to make sure you are using up at least 1000 calories a week. Gradually increase your activity level to 1500 and, finally, to 2000 calories a week.

The goal for everyone should be to double the amount of calories burned from exercise. If you start at 500, reach for 1000; 750, go for 1500; 1000, head for the "gold," or 2000 calories a week. Remember, you don't have to reach your goal overnight. It should take several weeks to go from your starting point to a level that is double that amount.

It's easier than you think to burn calories by moving. You can use up 1,000 a week by playing nine holes of golf, taking 3 half-hour walks and gardening for 2 hours. Mix and match activities you enjoy—even housework counts!

See Appendix 1 for your Weekly Activity Log and the chart Using Up Calories Through Activity.

Your activity goal is to burn ____ calories each week.

Goal: Work toward accomplishing the initial activity goal you've set. Every 2 to 3 weeks, as your stamina and fitness increase, set a new goal for yourself by adding more activity to burn up more calories. Your ultimate goal is to burn up double the amount of calories you set as your initial goal.

Now You're on Your Way to Success

We know that we've asked you to work very hard in this chapter, but it's worth it. Self-analysis is an important step toward self-awareness, which is necessary before behavior can be effectively changed. You are about to begin changing your eating and activity habits to achieve a slimmer, healthier you. So let's get started!

Chapter 9, **Smart Start**, offers you instant success. Follow the 28-day eating plan plus your individualized exercise plan and watch the weight drop off. Whether you need to lose a little or a lot to reach your target weight, **Smart Start** is a good place to begin.

It is hard to change lifestyle habits overnight. We give you a hand in **Smart Start** by planning your meals—you work on the rest. Many of our clients like this approach. You don't need to do all the work, at first, and you still get results. If you want to lose 5 to 15 pounds, **Smart Start** will get you to your target weight quickly.

If you need to lose more than 15 pounds, **Smart Start** helps you achieve some weight loss right away. Some of our clients like to stay on this 28-day eating plan for two or even three cycles. You may, too.

After **Smart Start** you'll move to Chapter 10, **Moving Along.** At this point, *you'll* plan what you eat each day. You can continue on this phase of *Get Skinny* until you've reached your target weight. Some of our clients, who only want to lose 5 to 7 pounds, prefer to begin with Chapter 10, **Moving Along**. That's an option, too. The whole idea of *Get Skinny the Smart Way* is to individualize it into *Your Personalized Weight Attack Plan.*

Once you've reached your target weight, the material in Chapter 11, **You're in Control**, will ensure that you do not regain the weight you've lost.

And remember, everything you've learned and every behavior change you've made is now part of your own personalized program to prevent gaining weight again. If you ever face a stressful time in your life or you find your weight creeping up again, go back to **Smart Start** or **Moving Along** and boost your resolve to eat well, exercise and take good care of yourself.

Chapter 8

A Closer Look at Food

Since food is the only source of body substance, persistent overfeeding is the only way to gain weight.

—Mary Swartz Rose, Ph.D., 1919

In this chapter you'll be taking a closer look at food. You'll examine options in every situation where you have to face food and decide what to do—when you shop, when you eat out, when you travel and during those loved, but dreaded, holiday meals.

Nutrients, Nutrients, Nutrients

In a word, that is why food is so important. It provides you with the more than 40 necessary nutrients you need to be healthy. Relax, we're not going to put you to work keeping track of all 40. We just want you to realize how important it is to make good food choices. After all, you are what you eat.

WHEN YOU SHOP

Supermarkets are moving from the business of selling individual foods to selling meals.

Lowfat, no fat, light, lean, sugar-free—which is best? You're told to "eat more fruits and vegetables," but they may come covered with buttery, cheesy or sugary sauces. You're told to "eat more carbohydrates," so you load up on sugar, white bread and pasta instead of whole grains.

Picking good food can be confusing. Even though the average supermarket stocks over 15,000 foods, along with another 15,000 nonfood items, most people eat only 35 different foods in any given week. It's hard to choose from the huge number of foods available given the limited time you have to shop, and the fact that you need to consider likes and dislikes of the people you live with.

You get home from work, the house is messy, the kids have homework, you forgot to pick up the clothes from the cleaner, you need to drive someone somewhere and everyone wants to eat right now. The first order of business is to get dinner on the table. This takes, in the average house, about eighteen minutes. At the same time, a voice in your head keeps reminding you that you're trying to cut calories. How do you manage to get everything done? *Get Skinny the Smart Way* offers many simple shortcuts that will help.

In this chapter we're going to take a closer look at food. We can't give you all the answers because food products appear and disappear all the time.

And your complicated life must be considered along with your diet plan. We'll arm you with information you can use to make the best choices while saving time putting together tasty, healthy meals that won't sabotage your weight loss goals.

Smart Shopping

Smart shopping strategies will help you navigate the food market so you'll leave with a supply of food that will help keep you, and those you live with, healthy while you eat the foods you need to reach your target weight.

- Don't go food shopping on an empty stomach.
  When you're hungry you buy more food than you actually need.

- Know the layout of the store where you shop.

  This saves time and cuts down on spontaneous buying.
- Products at eye level sell better than those shelved above or below.

  Bending and reaching not only burns calories but may also offer you better choices for less money.
- Make a list before you shop.

  This ensures you'll only buy those foods that fit into your diet plan. But you should allow yourself one impulse item per trip.
- Large is not always a better value.

  A bargain-size container is good only if you'll use it before it spoils. A half-gallon of milk costs less than two quart containers, but can you drink that much before the milk sours?
- Single servings save calories.

  Individually packaged fruit, ice cream, pudding, chips, cookies, cereal and yogurt are an easy way to eat common-sense portions.
- Money-off coupons tempt you to buy items you wouldn't ordinarily use.

  Cutting down on impulse purchases cuts down extra calories.
- Be an assertive shopper.

  Ask for assistance and insist on service. When the amount is too much, don't be afraid to ask for less. Request half a cabbage or melon, ask for a package with a quarter pound of ground turkey or one boneless chicken breast.

Get Skinny's
Smart Food Choices

Use This	Instead of This
Breads, Cereals, Grains	
Whole wheat bread	White bread
Whole wheat cereals (oatmeal, Wheatena, grape-nuts)	Cereals with little or no fiber

Use This	Instead of This
Raisin bread	Raisin cookies
Popcorn, plain	Popcorn, buttered
Pretzels	Potato chips
Angelfood cake and chocolate syrup	Chocolate cake with chocolate icing
Graham crackers	Cookies
Plain bagel	Croissant

Milk, Yogurt, Cheese, Ice Cream

Nonfat or reduced fat milk	Whole milk
Nonfat or reduced fat yogurt	Whole milk yogurt
Reduced fat cheese	Whole milk cheese
Reduced-calorie ice cream, sorbet, ices, frozen yogurt	Premium ice cream
Fudgesicles	Chocolate ice cream
Flavored nonfat milk	Milkshake

Vegetables, Fruits

Romaine, escarole, radicchio, Chinese cabbage	Iceberg lettuce, Belgian endive
Fresh fruit, fruit in juice or light syrup	Fruit in heavy syrup
Plain vegetables	Vegetables in butter, cream or cheese sauce
100% fruit juice	Juice drinks, punch, cocktail
Grapes	Raisins
Baked potato	French fries

Meat, Fish, Poultry

Flank steak	Short ribs
Lean hamburger or ground turkey	Regular hamburger
Pork tenderloin	Spareribs
Canadian bacon, turkey bacon	Bacon
Baked chicken	Fried chicken
Roast turkey	Self-basting roast turkey
Reduced-calorie beef or poultry hot dog	Beef hot dog
Grilled fish	Breaded fried fish
Sardines in mustard sauce	Sardines in oil

(continued)

Get Skinny's
Smart Food Choices (cont.)

Use This	Instead of This
Meat, Fish, Poultry (cont.)	
Tuna in water	Tuna in oil
Hard-cooked egg	Deviled egg
Fat free refried beans	Refried beans
Add-ons	
Nonfat cooking spray	Oil
Reduced-calorie salad dressing	Salad dressing
Fat free sour cream	Sour cream
Reduced-calorie or whipped cream cheese	Cream cheese
Whipped margarine or spray margarine	Stick margarine
Whipped butter	Stick butter
Reduced-calorie whipped topping	Whipped cream
Chocolate syrup	Hot fudge

SMART STUFF

Supermarkets are set up to encourage you to buy more. Milk is often at the rear of the store, so that as you walk through the store to get milk, you can be tempted to buy items you don't need.

Smart Selections

Ready-to-Eat Meals

What's for dinner? The quickest way to get food on the table might be a ready-to-eat dinner. Instead of cooking—just heat and eat. Use a stir fry frozen entrée, a bag of salad, brown-and-serve rolls, and individual pudding cups for dessert. Ready-to-heat-and-eat meals are planned for busy people.

On *Your Personalized Weight Attack Plan,* you'll be eating commonsense portions. Yet a study by the American Institute for Cancer Research found that only 12% of shoppers used the nutrition label to determine portion size. Zero in on portion size and the number of calories per portion. This will let you compare the food you're buying with the commonsense portions we recommend.

Many of the meals you buy suggest a 1 cup portion, less than you would probably eat. You'll need to do a little math to compare this to the more reasonable commonsense portions suggested in *Get Skinny.* For example, a *Get Skinny's* commonsense portion of pasta is 2 cups for a total of 400 calories. Any pasta meal you buy should not have more than 400 calories in a 2-cup portion. At first it will take a little time to read labels. But as you narrow down the best choices, the time you spend will be rewarded in calories saved.

SMART STUFF—Dates count

As little as 5% of shoppers pay attention to dates on food packages. Dates provide an excellent guide to freshness. If a *sell by* date is too close to the time of purchase, be sure you'll use the food up in a short time. Milk often has a *sell by* date. *Use by* dates give you an idea of how long a food can be kept and still be fresh. Most cereals have *use by* dates.

Bread, Cereals, Grains

Get Skinny*'s Commonsense Portions—*

Bread, Cereal, Pasta, Rice, Beans and Other Carbohydrate-Dense Foods

page 64

Your Personalized Weight Attack Plan encourages you to eat fiber-rich whole grains, which will help you lose weight faster. Experts urge us to eat whole grains, but most Americans still rely on white flour products for the majority of their choices.

Check the ingredient label to see if whole grains have been used. Bread labeled 100% whole wheat contains only whole wheat flour. Other whole grains—oatmeal, cracked wheat or rye—add fiber, too. Sometimes bread is made with more than one grain or a combination of whole grain and white flours. Other times the color can fool you. Some breads may look toasty brown and even be labeled "wheat," but that is from added caramel coloring, raisin juice or molasses, not whole wheat flour.

Today tortillas, bagels, croissants, muffins, pita and wraps are replacing old-fashioned sliced bread. Whole wheat versions are often available. Croissants and muffins are high in calories. Save them to be eaten once-in-a-blue moon.

Cereals, hot and cold, are not just for breakfast anymore. They fill you up, are rich in nutrients, and are usually low in fat. Unsweetened, high fiber cereals are the best, but are not always our first choice. Americans love sweetened cereal. As long as you stick with a commonsense portion—1 cup—sweetened cereal isn't off limits on the *Get Skinny* diet. Try mixing a sweetened cereal with a high fiber one. You can even enjoy a commonsense portion of cereal with added fruit or nuts.

Packages of instant hot cereals—oatmeal, Cream of Wheat, grits—come in many flavors, are portion controlled, moderate in calories, quick to prepare, and easy to keep on hand at home or in your desk drawer or locker at work. For a calcium boost, make the cereal with nonfat milk instead of water.

Cereals also make a good snack. If you crave peanut butter or chocolate, try a cereal flavored with your favorite flavor. Keep a commonsense portion in a reclosable bag in your handbag or desk drawer. It's a great low-calorie substitute for cake, cookies or candy when you want something sweet. When the coffee cart comes by, skip the chocolate muffin, have chocolate cereal instead. This switch could save 200 calories or more.

SMART STUFF

Instead of cake, try a waffle sundae. Top a toaster waffle with fruit and a spoonful of reduced-calorie whipped topping.

Quick and Easy Grain Recipes

Most people like white rice, but don't limit yourself. Try brown rice, barley, cornmeal, bulgur, kasha (buckwheat groats), pasta, and couscous. All of these have easy-to-follow cooking directions on the label and many come in quick-cooking varieties.

Brown rice, with more fiber, hasn't had its light brown coating removed. It cooks as quickly as white rice if you soak it first (see tip below) or use the quick-cooking or instant variety.

Tasty Rice—White or Brown

Follow package directions, but substitute tomato juice, vegetable juice or broth for water.

Brown Rice Risotto

Coat a frying pan with olive oil-flavored nonstick cooking spray. Cook 1 cup of quick cooking or presoaked brown rice and 1 chopped onion for 4 minutes. Add 1 can (14 ounces) fat free chicken broth and ¼ cup water, bring to a boil. Reduce heat to low and cook until broth is absorbed, about 15 minutes. Mix in 1 tablespoon of grated parmesan cheese and ¼ teaspoon black pepper.

1 serving = 1 cup   179 calories

Time Saving Tip—Soaking brown rice in water overnight or for several hours shortens the cooking time to only 20 minutes.

Spicy Rice and Beans

Prepare 1⅓ cups instant brown rice according to package directions. Stir in 1 can (15 ounces) red beans (drained and rinsed) and ½ cup salsa. Serve on a bed of lettuce.

1 serving = 1 cup   170 calories

Confetti Couscous

Couscous, available regular or whole wheat, takes only 10 minutes to prepare.

Mix 1 cup couscous with 1 can (14 ounces) fat free chicken broth and ¼ cup water, simmer five minutes. Add ½ cup each frozen corn and peas, and ½ to 1 teaspoon curry powder during the last 3 minutes of cooking.

1 serving = 1 cup   173 calories

Mediterranean Bulgur Salad

Bulgur is cracked wheat that cooks quickly.

Add 2 cups boiling water to 1 cup bulgar, stir, cover and let sit for 20 minutes. Add 1 cup cubed cucumber, 1 diced tomato, ¼ cup chopped, fresh parsley (or 1 teaspoon dried) and 1 to 2 tablespoons lemon juice (to taste). This salad can do double duty as a side dish or sandwich filling for a pita.

1 serving = 1 cup   87 calories

Kasha Delight

Kasha, also called buckwheat groats, is a nutty, rich brown grain that's also quick-cooking.

Heat a nonstick frying pan over moderate heat and add 1 cup kasha. Stir in 1 beaten egg, cook until dry—a minute or two. Reduce heat to low. Add 2½ cups water and ¼ teaspoon salt. Cover and cook for 10 minutes until water is absorbed. Just before serving, stir in I can (14 ounces) flavored, diced tomatoes.

1 serving = 1 cup   159 calories

Old-Fashioned Rice Pudding

Old-Fashioned Rice Pudding is easy to make, delicious and loaded with calcium that helps you lose weight.

Combine ½ cup uncooked rice and 3 cups nonfat milk in a heavy pan. Cook covered on low heat, stirring occasionally, for

30 minutes or until rice is soft. Add ⅓ cup sugar and 1 teaspoon vanilla. Add 1 slightly beaten egg and cook, stirring constantly for 2 minutes until thickened.

1 serving = ½ cup   157 calories + 140 milligrams calcium

Cooking Tip: If you are a lemon lover, omit vanilla and add the grated rind of ½ lemon plus 1 tablespoon lemon juice.

Milk, Yogurt, Cheese, Ice Cream

Get Skinny the Smart Way
recommends
2 servings of lowfat, calcium-rich foods
+ a 600 milligram calcium supplement daily

People have gotten the message that nonfat and reduced-fat milk and other dairy products are the best sources of calcium. Sales of nonfat milk have tripled in the last decade. Getting enough calcium helps you stay healthy and win the weight war. People with the lowest calcium intakes are six times more likely to be overweight. Calcium is a powerful dieting ally.

Getting enough calcium reduces body fat. But that's not all—we need plenty of calcium to keep our bones strong, help control high blood pressure, reduce premenstrual syndrome (PMS), and help prevent colon cancer and kidney stones.

Nonfat and reduced-fat milk, nonfat and reduced fat yogurt, and reduced fat cheese are readily available and are some of your best calcium sources. They contain all the calcium and other nutrients found in the regular varieties but with less calories.

SMART STUFF

It may sound old-fashioned, but lowfat evaporated milk is a creamy, low calorie substitute for cream in your coffee; 25 calories instead of 80 in 2 tablespoons.

Boxed, shelf stable milk is available in stores and can stay in the kitchen cabinet for as long as 6 months. Shelf stable yogurt is a good calcium-rich food to keep in your desk drawer.

Stirring 1 to 3 teaspoons of pectin into a container of yogurt creates an instant hunger chaser. Blending fruit—bananas, applesauce, berries—into the yogurt-pectin mix makes a luscious breakfast smoothie. Or you can stir pectin into a glass of calcium-rich instant breakfast drink to make you feel fuller longer.

Many fruit juices, soy milks, cereals, and desserts have extra calcium added. Adding a tablespoon of nonfat dry milk to a serving of cooked cereal, mashed potatoes, soup, instant pudding, creamy salad dressing, vegetables with sauce and other foods you make at home is another way to boost your calcium intake.

Canned salmon and sardines, with their soft bones, are other good sources of calcium. So are green, leafy vegetables like spinach, broccoli and kale. The calcium in vegetables comes packaged with very few calories so you can eat more. In Chapter 5 we gave you a list of traditional sources of calcium. Following are some others that might surprise you. With all these choices, it's easy to eat the recommended 2 servings of calcium-rich food each day.

Some Surprising Sources of Calcium

Food	Amount	Milligrams of Calcium
Almonds	¼ cup	79
Baked beans	1 cup	140
Broccoli	1 cup	94
Cheese pizza	1 slice	220
Frozen yogurt	½ cup	130
Ice cream	½ cup	100
Macaroni and cheese	1 cup	200
Tofu	4 ounces	164
Tomato soup	1 cup	160

Choosing a Calcium Supplement

The *Get Skinny* diet recommends taking a 600 milligram supplement each day to get the rest of the calcium you need. The most commonly available supplement is calcium carbonate, usually made from oyster shells. It is well absorbed, inexpensive, and the pills are small enough to be swallowed easily. Calcium citrate malate and calcium gluconate are other choices. These are bulkier and may be harder to swallow. Calcium chews are also available. Experts suggest taking calcium supplements at bedtime because the calcium is better absorbed while you sleep. Eating calcium-rich foods throughout the day, and taking a supplement in the evening increases absorption.

SMART STUFF

Adequate vitamin D is needed to absorb calcium. Studies show that significantly overweight people tend to have low levels of vitamin D in their blood. You get the vitamin from sun exposure and from fortified milk and cereals.

Vegetables and Fruits

Get Skinny's Commonsense Portions—

Vegetables and Fruits

page 70

There are over 400 fruits and vegetables, many of which are available year round. But with all the variety, surveys show the top selling vegetables are potatoes, lettuce, tomatoes, onions and carrots. Don't stick to the ones you always buy. When you shop, look over the produce. If you come across an unfamiliar vegetable or fruit, ask the produce manager what it is and how to use it.

Ready-to-eat fruits and vegetables—cut-up melons, sliced pineapples, fresh fruit salads, celery and carrot sticks, cut-up vegetables, and mixed salad greens are widely available. They make it easier for you to prepare meals. In 1999, over 90% of shoppers purchased fresh-cut salads and salad mixes. Many stores also offer well-stocked salad bars for a build-your-own salad.

Build a Better Salad—No Knife Needed

- The foundation of most salads is lettuce.

   Iceberg is crunchy and has a long refrigerator life, but it comes with few vitamins. Try less familiar, vitamin-rich romaine, escarole, endive, spinach, and cabbage—the deeper the green, the more vitamin-rich the variety.
- Add 4 or more of the following for flavor, color and nutrients.

   Cucumbers, tomatoes, red, green or yellow peppers, green beans, zucchini, carrots, mushrooms, cauliflower, broccoli, radishes, and scallions—the list goes on and on. New additions are constantly popping up. Edamame (fresh, green soybeans) are a tasty new addition to the salad bowl.
- Try fruits.

   Orange sections, apples, pears, grapes and melon cubes can be added to salads for a change of pace.
- Go easy.

   Olives, croutons, cheese, marinated vegetables, and oil add flavor but also add calories.
- For a flavor punch.

   Try roasted red peppers, grilled vegetables, artichoke hearts, mushrooms in vinegar, and cracked pepper.
- For a fiber boost.

   Add any kind of cooked, canned beans.
- Salad dressings are not off limits; look for reduced calorie choices.

   Try a few of the reduced-flavor choices to find your favorite. Pick those with no more than 80 calories in 2 tablespoons. Flavored vinegars are a nice change. Try adding buttermilk or nonfat yogurt to make any dressing creamy with fewer calories.

- Turn a salad into a meal.

    Add cooked, canned beans, sliced egg, tuna or leftover meat or poultry.

Though you often hear "fresh is best," frozen and canned fruits and vegetables are good choices, too. They are picked ripe and processed on the spot to lock in freshness. All vegetables and fruits are best "naked." Dressed with cheese sauce, butter, or sugary syrups, they quickly add on calories.

SMART STUFF

It may be hard to believe, but cooked vegetables are better than raw ones at protecting you against cancer and heart disease. Cooking releases antioxidants that fight tissue damage and the accumulation of plaque in arteries. You absorb five times more antioxidants when vegetables are cooked.

Fruit can serve as a snack, dessert, special breakfast treat or as the basis of a meal replacement in a glass. The following recipes will help you be more inventive with fruits.

Blueberry Pectin Smoothie

In a food processor or blender, combine ½ cup nonfat vanilla yogurt, ⅓ cup frozen or fresh blueberries, ⅓ cup bananas and 1 tablespoon pectin. Process until smooth.

Makes 1 single serving   226 calories

Fruit Smoothie

In a food processor or blender, combine ½ cup seedless grapes, ½ cup strawberries, ½ sliced banana and ½ sliced orange. Process until smooth. For a hunger chaser, stir in 1 to 3 teaspoons of pectin.

Makes 1 single serving   117 calories

High Energy Drink

In a food processor or blender, combine ½ cup soy milk, 1 cup of fruit, frozen or fresh (peaches, strawberries, pineapple, melon), ½ cup juice (orange, carrot, cranberry), and 1 tablespoon honey. Process until smooth.

1 serving = 2 cups   234 calories

Pineapple Slush Cocktail

These refreshing drinks are favorites in Jamaica.

In a food processor or blender, combine 1 cup of fresh pineapple, 2 tablespoons lemon juice, 1 tablespoon sugar, 1 cup crushed ice. Process for 1 minute. Makes 2 cups.

1 serving = 1 cup   64 calories

Baked Apple

Core an apple and place it in a small microwave baking dish. Fill the apple cavity with 1 tablespoon apricot all fruit spread, 1 tablespoon raisins and a pinch of cinnamon. Microwave on high for 3 to 5 minutes or until the apple is tender.

Makes 1 serving   143 calories

Glazed Pineapple

1 fresh pineapple, peeled and cored
½ teaspoon cinnamon
¼ cup brown sugar
8 maraschino cherries

Spray a baking pan with nonstick cooking spray. Slice pineapple into 8 slices and place on baking pan. Combine the cinnamon and brown sugar, sprinkle over slices. Place a cherry in the center of each slice. Broil 2 minutes until sugar is bubbly and pineapple is warm. Makes 4 servings.

1 serving = 2 slices   135 calories

Tip: Peeled, cored pineapple is available in most supermarkets, making preparation even quicker.

Peach Sundae

Instead of peach pie a la mode—

Place a crumbled graham cracker in a dessert dish. Place a peach half (in light syrup) on the graham cracker, top with ½ cup frozen vanilla yogurt and ¼ cup frozen sweetened blueberries or raspberries.

Makes 1 serving   219 calories

Tip: Traditional peach pie à la mode has 479 calories. You just saved 260 calories.

Hold the Juice

More fruits and vegetables, less juice is a thin habit. Vegetable juices and fruit juices are good sources of vitamins and minerals, but they contain little fiber making them calorie dense and less satisfying to eat. Until you reach your target weight it's smarter to "chew" than "drink" your favorite.

> ## SMART STUFF—100% is best
> After you reach your target weight, it's okay to drink juice. Choose 100% juice. Calcium-fortified is an added bonus. Don't confuse 100% juice with fruit drinks, cocktails and punches that contain added water and sugar.

Meat, Fish, Poultry

Get Skinny's Commonsense Portions—
Meat, Fish, Poultry—4 ounces
page 68

Get Skinny's commonsense portion, 4 ounces, is about the size of a computer mouse. That's plenty, even though it's probably less than you usually eat. Lean fresh fish, meat and chicken are all readily available, as are ready-to-heat-and-eat choices. Marinated, prepared and ready-to-cook chicken and fish, can be found in most stores. Some meat, fish and poultry is calorie dense because of added fat, breading, cheese, or sauce. Compare the calories in a portion on the nutrition label with *Get Skinny*'s commonsense portions.

The news has reported many stories about meat and poultry that have caused people to become ill. Most of these foodborne illnesses are minor but some can be serious. The best way to ensure your food is safe is to cook it to the correct temperature and check it with a kitchen thermometer. Instant-read thermometers make this easy.

Temperature Rules*

Food	Cook to °F
Ground Meat and Meat Mixtures	
Beef, pork, veal, lamb	160
Turkey, chicken	165
Fresh Beef, Veal, Lamb	
Medium rare	145
Medium	160
Well done	170
Fresh Pork	
Medium	160
Well done	170

*Food Safety and Inspection Service, United States Department of Agriculture, Washington, D.C., 20250–3700, www.fsis.usda.gov, Meat and Poultry Hotline: 1–800–535–4555

Food	Cook to °F
Poultry	
Chicken and turkey, whole	180
Poultry breasts, roast	170
Poultry thighs, wings	180
Duck and goose	180
Stuffing (cooked alone or in bird)	165
Ham	
Fresh (raw)	160
Pre-cooked (to reheat)	140
Egg and Egg Dishes	
Eggs	Cook until yolk and white are firm
Egg dishes	160
Leftovers and casseroles	165

SMART STUFF—Flip for safety

Cooking meat well done causes the formation of heterocyclic amines (HCA), substances that have been linked to an increased risk of cancer. A study reported in the *Journal of the National Cancer Institute* found that turning meat patties every minute during grilling or frying, greatly reduced the formation of HCA. Patties turned only once had higher levels of HCA.

Oven Roasted Pork or Beef Tenderloin

Roast a 1 pound boneless tenderloin at 425° F for 25 to 30 minutes. Add microwave baked potatoes and ready-to-use bagged salad to complete the meal.

1 serving = 4 ounces   185 calories for pork
258 calories for beef

Smart Leftovers: Thinly slice the leftover cooked meat and marinate it in 2 tablespoons light soy sauce and 2 tablespoons orange juice for 5 minutes. Prepare a package of your favorite vegetable combination, drain. Add sliced meat and marinade to vegetables and heat through. Serve over brown rice.

Spicy Fish

Divide one pound of your favorite fish fillets into 4 pieces. Place each piece on a square of foil and top with ¼ cup salsa, parsley and a squeeze of lemon juice. Fold the foil around the fish into packets and place on a baking sheet. Bake for 10 to 12 minutes at 400° F.

1 serving = 4 ounces   120 to 240 calories per serving, depending on the type of fish you select*

Lemon Fish Steaks

Place 1 pound fillet of cod, salmon or halibut (¾ to 1 inch thick) in a frying pan. Cover with water seasoned with ½ teaspoon dried or 1 fresh sprig dill, ½ teaspoon cracked pepper and a few lemon slices. Bring the flavored water to a boil. Turn off the heat, cover the pan, letting the fish finish cooking in the hot water for 8 to 10 minutes or until it flakes.

1 serving = 4 ounces   120 to 240 calories per serving, depending on the type of fish you select*

SMART STUFF

Eating more fish may help relieve depression and moodiness. Fish is loaded with omega-3 fatty acids that help your body regulate serotonin, a substance that lifts your spirits. Albacore tuna and salmon have high levels of omega-3 fatty acids. Two servings a week can improve your mood.

---

*See Commonsense Portions: Meat, Fish and Poultry, page 68 or Appendix 3, Keeping Track of What You Eat, page 332, for calorie values.

Orange Chicken & Vegetables

Prepare a package of stir-fry vegetables according to directions. Combine 2 tablespoons soy sauce and 2 tablespoons orange marmalade. Add sauce and a 10-ounce package of ready-to-eat, sliced chicken. Heat for 1 minute more. Makes 4 servings.

1 serving = approximately 170 calories,
depending on vegetable choice.

Serving Tip: Serve over cooked soba noodles.

Mustard Chicken Breasts

Coat a baking pan with nonstick cooking spray. Place 4 chicken breasts on the pan. If they are large, cut them in half. Coat the tops with your favorite mustard and sprinkle each with 1 tablespoon seasoned bread crumbs, and some parsley. Bake at 375° F for 15 to 20 minutes or until chicken is cooked through.

1 serving = 1 chicken breast   197 calories

SMART STUFF

Tofu, made from soy milk, has as much protein as meat. You can buy flavored, seasoned or reduced fat brands. Some come already cooked or marinated. Because tofu is naturally mild tasting, it soaks up flavors from other ingredients. The firmer the tofu, the better it holds its shape. Try stir-frying firm tofu with vegetables flavored with teriyaki sauce for a simple, nonmeat meal.

Smothered Sausage & Onion

Coat a frying pan with nonfat cooking spray. Brown 1 pound of lowfat chicken or turkey sausage for 3 to 4 minutes. Remove sausages from the pan. Add 1 teaspoon oil, 2 onions chopped and 2 cloves chopped garlic. Cook until onions are soft and lightly browned. Slice the sausages and return to the onion mixture, cooking 2 to 3 minutes more.

Makes 4 servings   1 serving = 219 calories

Serving Tip: Serve over cooked rice or pasta.

A Word About Eggs

Eggs have gotten a bad rap in recent years which is a shame, because they are nutritious and a good dieting choice. A hard-boiled egg (80 calories) is portable and versatile. Try a sliced-egg sandwich topped with 1 tablespoon salsa and crunchy lettuce on whole wheat bread; lunch for less than 300 calories. Enjoy a cup of green tea along with the sandwich to help burn calories and fat.

Lightly coating a frying pan with nonfat cooking spray is a perfect way to cook a scrambled egg. Add some toast and half a grapefruit and you have breakfast. Change a side salad to a lunch salad by topping with a sliced hard-boiled egg. Add a few bread sticks and you have a meal. Hard cook a half dozen eggs to have on hand. They'll keep in the refrigerator for a week.

If your doctor has told you to watch your cholesterol, try cholesterol-free egg substitutes. These can be used in place of whole eggs or used to stretch eggs. For people with normal cholesterol levels, it's really okay to eat an egg a day.

Let's Face Fats

Most experts agree—less fat is better. Foods high in fat are calorie dense. Eating too much fat will make you fatter faster. Yet most of us get over a third of our calories from fat. Foods high in fat are tempting and pack a lot of calories into a small portion. Fats have more than twice the calories in proteins and carbohydrates.

1 teaspoon of fat = 45 calories

1 teaspoon of carbohydrate (starch or sugar) = 20 calories

1 teaspoon of protein = 20 calories

Choosing Fats

Corn, canola, olive, peanut, safflower, cottonseed, and vegetable oils are all on the supermarket shelf. Oils are liquid fats used in cooking. Extra virgin olive oil has the strongest flavor. When baking or making desserts, oils with a bland taste like corn, canola, vegetable or light, mildly flavored olive oil are best.

Solid shortenings are made from liquid oils that have been processed to "harden" the oil. When this is done, some of the unsaturated fats, naturally found in oil, become *trans* fatty acids. Trans fats act like saturated fats and can raise cholesterol. When you see the words *hydrogenated* or *partially hydrogenated* in the food's ingredient list, you'll know that the food contains some trans fatty acids. Many food manufacturers are limiting their use of trans fatty acids. Tub or liquid margarines are softer with fewer trans fats than stick margarines.

Reduce Fat, Reduce Calories

- Mist oil or measure it out; keep the amounts low.
- Butter sprinkles and sprays add flavor with few calories.

    Add butter sprinkles, instead of butter, to mixes like instant mashed potatoes and rice combos.

- You can sabotage a salad by adding too much dressing or grated cheese.

    Stick with commonsense portions: 2 tablespoons of dressing and 1 tablespoon of grated cheese.

- Use reduced-calorie salad dressing with no more than 80 calories in a 2 tablespoon commonsense portion.

    The range of calories in "reduced-calorie" dressings is enormous. Fat free dressings have 20 to 50 calories in 2 tablespoons. Light versions have 13 to 80 calories in 2 tablespoons. None are calorie-free.

    Using lemon juice or flavored vinegar (with 0 to 10 calories in a tablespoon) cuts calories the most.

- Whipped cream cheese, butter, margarine and whipped toppings all have fewer calories than the regular versions—

or—use light butter or margarines. The air whipped in to give them their light, fluffy texture eliminates some fat calories.

- Cut calories with nonfat yogurt.

    Added to mayonnaise, tartar sauce or regular salad dressing to make it creamy, you get the same taste with less calories.

- Use nonfat heavy cream and sour cream. These are lower calorie alternatives for coffee or a baked potato.

- Choose tuna in water with 7 times less calories than tuna in oil.

- Choose nonfat and reduced fat milk and cheese. They have the same calcium, protein and other nutrients with far less calories.

- Use lean cuts of meat and poultry and remove all the visible fat before you cook.

    Poultry skin is high in fat. You can cook poultry with its skin on, but remove it before eating. For even less calories, buy skinless or remove skin before cooking.

- Avoid turkey and turkey breasts that are self-basting. The basting adds fat calories.

- All varieties of fish contain less fat than most cuts of meat.

    The leanest choices are cod, scrod, flounder, halibut, pollock, sole, haddock, shrimp, lobster, scallops, mussels, and crab. Remove the skin from fattier fish like salmon, mackerel or bluefish.

- Broil, roast, grill, steam, stew or poach fish, poultry and lean meats. Frying, breading, batter and butter adds calories.

- Explore the supermarket's reduced fat foods. As long as you stick with a commonsense portion, they'll fit nicely into your *Get Skinny* diet.

Don't Forget Water

Your Personalized Weight Attack Plan recommends you drink 8 to 10 glasses of water or other liquids each day. Only about one third of us drink that much. When you drink too little your body burns calories less efficiently. Being well hydrated actually helps you use up calories faster.

People are very busy, often too busy to stop for a drink of water. Make it a habit to drink some water every couple of hours. Tap water is safe and healthy but many people prefer brand name bottled water. That's fine, but go easy on vitamin-fortified and caffeine-enhanced waters.

All juices, milk, and caffeine-free coffee, tea and soda count. Alcohol can't be counted as a source of water. But you can count half of the caffeine-containing coffee, tea, and soda you drink. Stay away from heavily sweetened drinks or soda because they are high in calories as well.

Green tea is a good way to get some fluids and it helps you burn calories and fat. Experts recommend green tea every day because of its high antioxidant content. We encourage you to drink at least a cup a day.

Flavor Boosters

Just Taste, No Calories

Balsamic vinegar—Adds tang to food. To make Balsamic Cucumber Salad, peel and thinly slice a cucumber into a small bowl. Add 2 teaspoons balsamic vinegar, ½ teaspoon sugar, salt to taste and a little chopped onion, if you like. Chill.

1 serving = 1 cup   50 calories

Cooking spray—Flavored sprays—butter, olive oil, garlic—can make a plain vegetable special. To make Microwave Tomatoes, slice 2 or 3 tomatoes into half-inch slices. Place on a microwave-safe baking dish. Coat the tomatoes lightly with your favorite spray. Microwave for 1–2 minutes until tomatoes are soft.

Cracked pepper—Freshly cracked pepper adds zest to food. Add a sprinkle on soups, vegetables, pasta and salads.

Flavored vinegar—As little as a teaspoon can add a spark of flavor to any dish. Add 1 teaspoon mustard, ½ teaspoon salt, ¼ teaspoon cracked pepper and 2 teaspoons olive oil to

¼ cup of your favorite flavored vinegar. Pour over cooked green beans, chill before serving.

Hot sauce—A couple of drops of hot sauce and some chopped onion added to lean, ground turkey, chicken, or beef will make burgers special.

Horseradish—Add a little grated horseradish to nonfat yogurt or ketchup and enjoy it as a robust topping for a sandwich, vegetables or fish.

Lemons—A wedge of lemon can make a glass of water or a cup of tea tangy. Grated lemon peel adds zest to stir-fries and a dash of lemon juice enhances the taste of fish. To make Lemon Ice, a low-calorie, refreshing snack, combine 1½ cups water and ½ cup sugar in a medium saucepan. Bring to a boil, simmer 5 minutes. Remove from heat. Stir in 3 ounces frozen, concentrated lemonade. Pour into a shallow, plastic dish and freeze for 1 to 2 hours, or until firm. Stir once or twice while ice is hardening.

1 serving = ½ cup   114 calories

Light soy sauce—All the flavor with half the salt of regular. To make Ginger Tofu, combine 2 tablespoons light soy sauce, 1 clove garlic, sliced (or ½ teaspoon garlic powder), 1 tablespoon red wine vinegar, and ¼ teaspoon ground ginger in a bowl. Slice 1 package (16 ounces) extra firm tofu into ¼-inch pieces. Add tofu to soy sauce mixture. Soak for 15 minutes and drain tofu. Broil tofu until lightly browned, about 2 minutes on each side. Makes 4 servings.

1 serving = 4 ounces   108 calories

Mustard—Explore the many textures and flavors of mustards. To make Mustard Pepper Beans, combine 1 tablespoon mustard, 1 tablespoon lemon juice, 2 tablespoons vinegar, and 2 tablespoons olive oil. Pour dressing over 1 (15 ounce) can beans (drained and rinsed) mixed with 1 cup diced red and yellow peppers.

1 serving = 1 cup   212 calories

Salsa—The nation's number one topper used, with sales outstripping the once favorite ketchup, it can be found in tomato, bean, peach, roasted pepper, corn, pineapple and artichoke flavors. To make Salsa Corn Salad combine ⅓ cup of your favorite with 1 medium chopped onion, 1 medium seeded and chopped green pepper, and 1 can (11 ounce) corn, drained. Serve over chopped romaine.

1 serving = 1 cup   71 calories

Worcestershire sauce—Adds color and flavor. To make Worcestershire Medley Pasta Sauce, finely chop 1 onion and 1 stalk of celery, combine with 1 cup grated carrots (about 2 carrots). Coat a frying pan with nonstick cooking spray and stir fry vegetables until they are soft. Add 2 cups of sliced mushrooms and continue cooking for 5 minutes. Stir in 2 teaspoons Worcestershire sauce and ¼ cup water. Simmer for 5 minutes. Serve over cooked pasta.

Makes 2 servings   1 serving = 105 calories (sauce) + 400 calories (2 cups pasta)

Lots of Taste, a Few Calories

Ketchup—An addition that makes (almost) everything taste better. It adds color and flavor to meat dishes, vegetables, even mashed potatoes.

All fruit jelly—Bread isn't the only food that tastes better with jelly. Try a spoonful of jelly on cooked cereal, pancakes, waffles or unsalted crackers. Try Broiled Grapefruit for a change at breakfast. Spread grapefruit half with 1 teaspoon of your favorite flavor all fruit jelly. Microwave for 30 seconds on medium.

1 serving = ½ grapefruit   69 calories

Reduced-calorie dressing—It's not just for salad. Dress your favorite sandwich or try some as a marinade for raw fish and chicken—it adds taste when grilling or broiling. Turn left-over vegetables into a veggie salad with a drizzle and some fresh onion slices.

Anchovy paste—Comes in a tube so you can squeeze out small amounts to add a subtle, pleasing flavor to soups and dips with only 14 calories in a teaspoon.

Sherry pepper—Combine ¼ cup chopped, fresh hot peppers and 1 cup cooking sherry (or table sherry, if you prefer). Store in a glass bottle (a leftover, washed vinegar, soy sauce or Worcestershire bottle works well). This interesting concoction will infuse a spirited taste into many foods without making the dishes hot. Try a little in tomato sauce, over grilled meats, in fried onions or add a bit to stir-fries.

WHEN YOU EAT OUT

On average, Americans eat out 18 times a month, spending one billion dollars a day in the process.

—Consumer Reports

In Chapter 6 we told you about thin habits you can use to enjoy an evening out that won't sabotage your weight loss goals. Rely on those behavioral changes when you eat away from home.

But modifying eating behavior is just one tool. You also need to know how to be an assertive customer. How to decipher the menu. What options to order in ethnic restaurants. And how to cope with snatch-and-grab, eat-on-the-run choices that make up the majority of your eating out experiences.

A restaurant meal used to be a much anticipated adventure. It happened so infrequently, it was okay to overdo. That's not the case anymore. In 1999, over a billion restaurant meals were ordered. Almost half of these were eaten at home but cooked in someone else's kitchen. In our time-compressed world, take-out has become a popular option. When you're eating out or ordering in, as often as we do today, you can't give yourself carte blanche to eat whatever you'd like.

On the contrary, it's more important to be vigilant about your eating behavior away from home because you have little control over the food's preparation. A study done at the University of Memphis and Vanderbilt University found that women who ate out more than 5 times a week ate almost 300 calories more a day, on average, than those who ate out less often. This adds up to a weight gain of 30 pounds in a year!

SMART STUFF

All-you-can-eat buffets can be a dieter's downfall. Studies show that the more foods people have to pick from the more they eat. Save buffets for once-in-a-blue-moon.

Let's Order

You walk into a restaurant, you're shown to a table and handed a menu. Believe it or not, your key to a successful evening of eating out while staying on target with your weight loss plan is right there in your hand. Reading the menu carefully and selecting the best choices is possible when you know key words and catch phrases to look for.

Menu selections with less calories and less fat are frequently listed as:

au jus (in its own juice)	grilled
baked	julienne
boiled	lean
broiled	marinara
cooked with lemon juice	poached
cooked with wine	roasted
deviled	steamed
fresh	stir fry
garden fresh	without skin

Menu choices that are more calorie dense should be reserved for once-in-a-blue-moon, ordered as a main dish in appetizer size, or split with a friend. These are usually described as:

au gratin	hash
battered	hollandaise
buttered	Kiev
breaded	parmesan
casserole	parmigiana
cheese sauce (Mornay)	pastry
cream sauce (à la king)	pot pie
creamy (Béchamel)	prime
creamed	rémoulade
crispy	rich
deep fried	scalloped
escalloped	thermidor
fried	
gravy	

If you are still working toward your target weight, hold off on these for a while.

Other menu items fall into the "ask about" category. Often the restaurant's version of this type of preparation will fit right into *Your Personalized Weight Attack Plan* as long as you stick with a commonsense portion.

à la grecque	vegetables cooked in lemon juice and some oil, which can be reduced
cacciatore	a chicken or fish sauce made with tomatoes, mushrooms and herbs
hunter sauce	brown sauce made with tomatoes, mushrooms and white wine
creole	spicy Southern sauce of tomato, pepper, and vegetables
scallopine	very thin slices of boneless meat or poultry, floured and sautéed in wine

SMART STUFF—Minus one
Restaurant meals are so large, a simple trick to cut back but still have enough to eat is to order 1 entrée less than the number in your party and share.

Some evenings the menu you're handed looks like it's written in a foreign language. It probably is if you are in one of the growing number of ethnic restaurants opening across the country. Even here, you can negotiate good choices.

In a Chinese Restaurant

Traditional Chinese and other Asian cuisines are quite healthy because most dishes are made with little meat and many vegetables. In the Americanized versions, the opposite is often true. The good news is that many dishes are "made to order," so you can request what you'd like. Ask for double vegetables in stir-fries. Order a serving of steamed vegetables to add to other dishes that are vegetable-less. Ask for green tea. Eat with chopsticks, it will make the meal last longer even if you're a pro.

Order This More Often	Than This
Steamed dumplings	Fried dumplings
Steamed wontons	Fried wontons
Clear soups	Egg drop soup
Rice, white or brown	Fried rice
Steamed noodles	Fried noodles or noodles in peanut sauce
Steamed egg rolls	Crispy egg rolls
Dim sum, steamed	Dim sum, fried
Steamed vegetable or tofu combos	Fried vegetable or meat combos
Stir-fries	Deep fried
Steamed combos	Combos with nuts
Steamed shrimp combos	Fried shrimp combos

(continued)

Once-In-A-Blue-Moon
Spareribs
Peking duck
Crispy chow mein noodles

In an Italian Restaurant

Pasta and pizza immediately come to mind. A commonsense portion of pasta is 2 cups, totaling 400 calories. Add to that oil, cheese, meat and you get the picture—many Italian meals are calorie dense. Today, many restaurants are adding lighter choices. Instead of butter, you can request a small dish of marinara sauce in which to "dip" bread. There are many things on an Italian menu you can eat if you're watching your calorie intake.

Order This More Often	Than This
Italian bread	Garlic bread
Grilled portobello mushrooms	Stuffed mushrooms
Minestrone soup	Lentil sausage soup
Tossed salad, dressing on the side	Caesar salad
Steamed artichoke	Stuffed artichoke
Spaghetti with garlic and oil	Fettuccini Alfredo
Marinara, pomodoro sauce	Carbonara, Bolognese or meat sauce
Clam sauce, white or red	Pesto
Pasta and beans	Pasta and meat or chicken
Pasta primavera	Pink sauce
Italian ice	Cannoli

Once-In-A-Blue-Moon
Cheese stuffed pasta
Lasagna
Parmigiana dishes
Stuffed crust pizza
Cheesecake

SMART STUFF—Just one slice

An average 4-ounce slice of cheese pizza has 300 calories. If you can eat just one, plus a tossed salad, no problem. Or, skip the cheese and try less calorie dense toppers: onions, mushrooms, green, red and yellow peppers, zucchini, eggplant, broccoli, tomatoes, roasted peppers, spinach, pineapple, ham, and Canadian bacon. Thin crust is best.

In a Middle Eastern Restaurant

Middle Eastern food can be Greek, Syrian, Lebanese, Turkish, Armenian or any combination. Many dishes are served with a drizzle of olive oil or topped with tahini (sesame seed butter) and whole milk yogurt sauce. But all can be left off or ordered on the side. Pita bread, cucumbers, couscous, rice pilaf and steamed vegetables are staples and great add-ons to any meal you choose.

Order This More Often	Than This
Hummus	Falafel
Baba ganoush	Fish roe dip
Stuffed grape leaves	Kasseri cheese casserole
Greek salad, dressing on the side	Taramolsalata
Lentil soup	Lemon soup
Cracked wheat salad	Spinach and feta cheese pies
Shish kebobs	Gyros
Marinated and grilled meat and chicken	Moussaka eggplant casserole
Kibbeh cracked wheat, meat and onions	Pasticchio macaroni and meat casserole

Once-In-A-Blue-Moon
Baklava pastry

In an Indian Restaurant

India is a huge country with a diverse cuisine. Restaurants in the U.S. feature food from every region. Some dishes are hot, some pungently sweet, others pickled, and curries are often a favorite. Food is often fried in ghee (clarified butter) and curries may be based in cream or coconut milk. Both can be omitted, if requested. Plain rice is a good staple.

Order This More Often	Than This
Lentil soups	Samosa
Chopped potato and tomato salad	Pakora
Chapati bread	Poori bread
Naan bread	Paratha fried bread
Tandoor clay baked	Korma creamed curry
Tikka, chicken or fish	Saag, chicken or lamb
Vindaloo, chicken, fish or beef	Masala, chicken, fish or beef
Raita cucumber sauce	Dahl lentil sauce
Chutney, mango or onion	Chutney, coconut

Once-In-A-Blue-Moon
Papadom fried wafers with dipping sauce

In a Mexican Restaurant

Mexican food is fast becoming one of the most popular ethnic dining choices. A bowl of tortilla chips and salsa usually greets you at the table. Skip the chips and ask for soft tortillas instead but enjoy as much salsa as you'd like.

Add-on's for dishes can add up. Skip shredded cheese, guacamole, and sour cream. But enjoy chopped onion, salsa, pico de gallo, red sauce and green sauce. Tostadas, burritos, enchiladas, and tacos all come stuffed. Select beans, chicken, shrimp, vegetables and chopped salad more often than beef, cheese and cream sauce.

Order This More Often	Than This
Vegetarian bean chili	Chili con carne with meat
Black beans	Refried beans
Soft tortillas	Crispy tortillas
Fajitas, chicken, beef or shrimp	Chimichanga or fried filled burrito
Chicken fajita salad	Beef taco salad

(continued)

Order This More Often	Than This
Arroz con pollo, chicken and rice	Flauta con crema, crisp stuffed tortilla with cream sauce
Soft stuffed taco	Fried stuffed tacos
Flan custard	Sopappillas fried dough

Once-In-A-Blue-Moon
Chicken or beef mole
Chili relleños

Don't Fall for the Subtle Sell

Waiters and waitresses are trained to "sell" you food. The good ones do it in such a charming, warm way you are unaware you're being pitched to buy something extra. "Can I get you anything from the bar while you look at the menu?" *Anything* could add up to a few hundred extra calories. Stick with water or sparkling water until you reach your target weight. If the table automatically comes stocked with foods you're trying to limit, ask that they be removed or request a substitute. "Could we have the bread basket, without the garlic bread?" Of course you can, if you ask.

"Our specials tonight are . . ." Specials are often made to order. This is a good opportunity to request that they be made to your order. Grilled not fried, light on the oil, gravy on the side or not at all, no cheese topping. Don't be afraid to be an assertive customer. You're paying for food and service, you should pay for what you want. But in all fairness to the restaurant, not all dishes can be modified. Have a second choice in case your first pick can't be made less calorie dense.

Think Before You Drink

Liquid calories don't register the same feeling of satisfaction but they can add up. Until you reach your target weight stick with no calorie drinks like water, sparkling water, mineral water, seltzer, diet soda, and unsweetened iced, green and herbal tea. *Curb calories in a glass* is a thin habit.

Even after you've reached your target weight, a simple way to eat less calories is to curb those extra calories you drink.

Order This More Often	Than This
Nonfat milk	Whole milk
Nonfat chocolate milk	Whole milk chocolate milk
Diet soda	Regular soda
Diet iced tea	Sweetened iced tea
Latte with skim milk	Latte with whole milk
Cappuccino with skim milk	Cappuccino with whole milk
Light beer	Regular beer
Merlot	Martini
White wine spritzer	White wine

SMART STUFF—Dilute alcohol

Alcohol packs a lot of calories into a small serving but you can make it less calorie dense. Turn wine into a spritzer with sparkling water or seltzer. Dilute hard liquor with fruit juice, tomato juice, and lots of ice.

On-the-Go Eating

You may not consider a stop at the doughnut shop eating out, but it is, and it counts. We've become a nation that eats on the run. Restaurants offer "drive-thrus," so you don't even need to leave the car. New cars are being designed with more cup holders and family vans are coming equipped with coolers. The thin habit, *eat at the table,* may be tough to practice.

We'd urge you not to eat "in motion" as often as you can but we also appreciate that "real life" must come first. If you have to eat on-the-go, we'll help you negotiate your way through the maze of temptations.

Doughnut shops, bagel stores, 24-hour quick-stops, pizza shops, luncheonettes, "drive-thrus," food courts at the mall, and food stands at the movies; this is a tough path to travel without yielding to temptation. Just knowing that temptation is lurking can be the first step to avoiding it.

You own tools and strategies that you can use in any eating situation. Every selection you are considering has a better option. Think small, half, share.

Order the smallest version of anything. Is half available? Many luncheonettes and food courts offer smaller portions of the regulars—a half sandwich and a cup of soup instead of a sandwich and chips with a bowl of soup. A short stack of pancakes, 2 instead of 4. Can you order the smaller luncheon portion even though it's dinner? Many places offer this option.

SMART STUFF—Ordering a diet plate?

Think twice. Not all "diet plates" are good for dieters. A typical coffee shop diet plate often features a 4-ounce lean beef patty, ½ cup of cottage cheese, a hard-cooked egg, tomato slices and "all you can eat" bread basket. This could add up to over 600 calories.

Sharing is a great way to spread calories around. Let the whole group share a slice of carrot cake with cream cheese frosting when you stop for coffee. Split an entrée and order a second salad. A buddy who will share is a good friend. A fellow dieter is a best friend.

SMART STUFF—Take the napkin test

When you think the food you picked has hidden calories, place it on a napkin. If it leaves a greasy ring, it has lots of fat calories. Blotting the top of food can have the same result. A greasy napkin = extra calories.

Many snacks, sandwiches, pastries—even chips and dip—are being packaged for one to eat on the run. Choose carefully. If labeled, check the calories per portion. Will that amount of calories fit into your target calorie zone? When there is no label, rely on your visual clues—yo-yo, computer mouse, tennis ball, Ping-Pong ball—to estimate the portion size. Is it commonsense size? If what you're holding isn't the best choice for *Your Personalized Weight Attack Plan,* look for an alternative.

Roadside restaurants offering value meals are tempting. "For only 25 cents you can add super fries to your order." The smiling counter person urges you to value-size your meal. Bigger isn't always better. It's not a bargain if you don't need it and you surely don't need extra calories while you're trying to lose weight. When you eat at a quick-service restaurant, pick menu items that are small and undressed.

SMART STUFF—Don't fall for fries

The value meal portion of French fries can have over 500 calories. If you can't resist, share a portion or order a kid-size. Americans love fries, we each eat 30 pounds a year.

WHEN YOU TRAVEL

550 million passengers board planes in the U.S. each year.

Eating in the Air

We're a country on the move for both work and pleasure. Many of you spend a lot of time in airports, waiting for connections, and on planes flying to your destination. Enroute you have to eat. Airport and airline fare has to fit into *Your Personalized Weight Attack Plan.* And it does.

The good news is that a recent survey by the American Dietetics Association showed that most airports are offering healthy food options. Overall, food selection has improved. Fresh fruit, fruit juices, bagels, pretzels, salads, and lowfat and nonfat yogurt (for a hunger chaser on-the-go) are all readily available. Some airports even have restaurants where you can customize a salad, sandwich or pasta dish.

For a double bonus, go for a walk around the airport to explore the eating options. This prevents you from grabbing the first thing you see and you'll be active at the same time. Airports today are enormous. If you walk from Terminal 1 to Terminal 3 at Chicago's O'Hare International Airport—the world's busiest— you'd travel over a mile. Dallas, Atlanta and other large city airports can easily become your indoor track. On a layover you can cover miles.

One of the best things about airline food is, good or bad, you get very little. Even a first class passenger is served commonsense portions. With long delays and hours sitting on the runway a possibility, packing survival rations in your carry-on or briefcase is wise. It will keep you from getting hungry and gorging on peanuts and chips, often the only options offered. Airlines have no regulations about passengers carrying their own food on the plane. In many cases picking up a good-for-you salad, before you board, may be better for your dieting goals than the unknown meal coming down the aisle.

SMART STUFF—Too heavy to take off

Even airlines have had to make adjustments for our nation-wide weight gain. By law, airplanes can't take off if they're too heavy. Everything on board must be calculated and the weight carefully distributed. For air travel safety the Federal Aviation Administration upgraded the standard weight figure they use for passengers when calculating the total weight on an aircraft.

Most airlines offer special meals if you request them a few days ahead of your flight or ask about them when you make your reservations. About 3% of passengers take advantage of this service. The most popular requests are "lighter" choices and vegetarian meals. Some airlines give passengers a choice between 2 or 3 meals. A survey showed that 60% of first class passengers and 70%

of coach passengers selected the more calorie dense breakfast when offered an option. You know better than that.

Sticking with your goal of drinking 8 to 10 glasses of water or other fluids daily is especially important when you fly. The low humidity and recirculating air in the pressurized cabin can be dehydrating and aggravates symptoms of jet lag, not to mention slowing down your ability to burn calories efficiently. Put some small bottles of water in your survival kit and be sure to drink at least 8 ounces for every hour you're on the plane, whether on the runway or in the air.

What to Eat When You Land

All the tips and strategies for eating out apply when you travel. Don't let a vacation or business trip derail your dieting goals. You can still try local specialties and enjoy regional cuisine, but too much of anything isn't a good idea. Stick with commonsense both in what you choose and how much you eat. This may be the time to declare a blue moon meal. But remember, blue moons don't happen regularly.

Business travelers often stay at the same hotel chain wherever they go. Take advantage of knowing the layout and facility. Use the gym or pool. If none are available, take a few laps around the enormous parking lot. Check to see if the hotel chain your company uses has a lighter fare option or can provide special meals for frequent visitors. Many do. To cut down on spontaneous snacking, don't accept the key to your room's mini bar.

Be selective if your hotel provides a complimentary breakfast. Many of the options are calorie dense. Many others—hot cereal, ready-to-eat cereal, nonfat milk, fresh fruit, whole wheat toast, yogurt—will fit right into *Your Personalized Weight Attack Plan*.

If you order room service, ask for just that, the service you need. You are paying a premium for these meals so you should get what you want. When you place your order ask for nonfat milk, whole wheat instead of white bread, an English muffin instead of pastry, extra vegetables, or low calorie salad dressing. By giving careful instructions to room service you can even order a **Smart Start** meal over the phone.

A Closer Look at Food—During the Holidays

Maintaining your weight during the holidays is an achievement to be applauded and a realistic goal.

Short of heading for a deserted island between Christmas and New Year's Day, what's the game plan for staying on a diet during the holidays? The game plan for *Get Skinny the Smart Way* never changes. That's why it works. Any time in any place that you face food there is a way to negotiate an option.

A recent study done in collaboration with the Medical University of South Carolina and the National Institutes of Health, showed that the typical holiday weight gain was little more than a pound, far less than most expected. The researchers concluded that the five-plus pounds people expect they'll gain is a myth. Appreciate that research indicates trends, not specifics, so if you use the holidays as an excuse, you could be the five-pound exception rather than the one-pound rule. The researcher also noted that even if the holiday weight gain is small, when it isn't lost in subsequent months it could become cumulative and, year after year, would be enough to account for "middle-age spread," ten pounds a decade.

The holidays are tough and while you may not lose as rapidly during them, you most definitely shouldn't gain.

If you host the party:

- Serve some lower calorie choices along with traditional dishes.
- Modify traditional recipes to be less calorie dense.
- Chew gum or plan a good-for-you nibble while you cook or bake.
- Give calories away—send your guests home with goodie bags.

When you're the guest:

- Before you go out, have a piece of fruit or a pectin hunger chaser to blunt your appetite.

- If you're looking forward to certain holiday food, plan ahead. Eat lighter during the day before the party or exercise more.
- Alternate drinks. Have one alcoholic or calorie dense drink, like eggnog, followed by two no-calorie drinks like diet soda or sparkling water with a twist of lemon.
- Dilute alcohol for more fluid and less calories per serving.
- Circulate away from the food and bar.
- Keep a beverage in one hand. It will be hard to hold a plate and eat with the other.
- Eat fewer fried and cheesy hors d'oeuvres; enjoy shrimp cocktail and cut-up fruits and veggies.
- Eat light at the meals before a party but don't fast or you'll feast.
- Exercise more the day before and after a holiday event.
- Survey the whole buffet table once, then get on line and make choosy choices.
- Want pie for dessert? Eat the filling, leave the calorie-dense crust. Pumpkin pie is such a healthy choice it can count toward your five-a-day fruits and veggies.
- Enjoy every meal, just don't supersize it.

SMART STUFF—Don't take the holidays lying down
After dinner, do the dishes, take a walk, play with the kids. Lying down or napping slows down the calories you burn and speeds up the possibility of heartburn.

Chapter 9

Smart Start

Hunger and satisfaction are simple words for a complex process that tells us when to eat and when to stop.

Getting started on a diet is hard—you feel like there are so many things you'll have to give up and so many things to change. The thought of it can be overwhelming.

We're aware of how you feel and that's why we developed **Smart Start**. It provides a structured beginning to *Get Skinny the Smart Way*. It takes some of the decisions out of your hands, until you're ready to take over. And it works.

We'll be a team for the next 28 days. We'll make most of the food decisions and you'll work on being more active. By relying on us you won't have to do everything.

And the best part—you'll lose weight quickly. This guaranteed quick success will give you the confidence to go further. Before you know it you'll have reached your target weight. You'll be in control.

Hungry? Full?

How do you know you're hungry?

How do you know when you've had enough to eat?

If eating were simply a matter of refueling our bodies when more energy was needed, life would be very simple. Feel hungry? Eat. Feel full? Stop. For most of us eating is far more complicated. Getting a handle on hunger and satisfaction can be powerful weapons in your own personal diet war.

Get Skinny's first thin habit is, *eat when you're hungry.* But we know that's not as easy as it sounds. Hunger can be defined as a group of subjective sensations you feel that motivates you to eat. Satisfaction refers to the sensations you feel that ends a meal. More simply put, hunger is the need for food and satisfaction is the result of having enough.

The problem with this simple explanation is that hunger and satisfaction mean different things to different people. Some people report "feeling" hunger in their stomachs, others in their head. Some claim it's a feeling of weakness and nausea. Others say they eat at certain times during the day, or when they see or smell food, without giving much thought to their body's signals.

Satisfaction after eating has equally varying descriptions—from a pleasurable sense of fullness, to a feeling of being stuffed, to the point of being uncomfortable and unhappy. Some eat until their plate is empty and declare themselves "finished and satisfied." Others eat so often or so much they never feel either hungry or satisfied. We want you to get a handle on both of these sensations.

That is part of the reason why **Smart Start** includes 3 meals and 3 snacks each day—to help you space out eating so you get tuned to your body's natural hunger cycle. Not eating when you are hungry or eating too much can disrupt the normal cues for hunger and satisfaction. Research has shown that even if our internal cues have been disrupted, they can be relearned. One way is to eat at normal intervals throughout the day. This gives your body a regular source of fuel with time between meals to use it up.

Another way to get in touch with your body is to rate the feeling of hunger before you eat and your satisfaction afterward. Using a five-point scale, consider 1 as not hungry and 5 as uncomfortably hungry. Use the same scale for satisfaction, 1 as not satisfied and 5 as uncomfortably full.

HUNGER SCALE

1	2	3	4	5
not hungry	a little hungry	hungry	very hungry	uncomfortably hungry

SATISFACTION SCALE

1	2	3	4	5
not full	somewhat full	satisfied	very full	uncomfortably full

You'll be surprised at how effective this simple exercise can be. It makes you stop and think about whether you are truly hungry and need food or whether you're just tempted to eat because you are stressed, bored, or see a delicious doughnut. The same holds true for your feelings of satisfaction. Many overweight people have lost touch with their sense of food satisfaction. If you almost always rate your sense of satisfaction as 4 (very full) or 5 (uncomfortably full), something other than food is causing you to eat. If you sometimes leave the table feeling 1 (not full), examine why. If you're not eating enough at meals, are you eating more at other times?

Social situations have a great deal to do with how much we eat. Eating behavior studies have shown people eat more with families than co-workers. They also eat more when presented with more choices, like a buffet. Meals high in carbohydrates, like pasta and potatoes, and low in fiber and protein, cause overeating. And the more you chew the less you eat. Sounds contradictory but it's true. Fluids (like soda) are less satisfying than semifluids (like soup), which in turn are less satisfying than solids (like a salad). The salad offers the most chewing. More chewing stretches out the time it takes to eat, giving your body time to register fullness and signal your brain to stop eating.

For the next 28 days, take a few seconds before and after you eat to rate your feelings of hunger and satisfaction. You'll begin to listen to your body and turn off the signals that have tempted you to eat too often or too much in the past.

Let's Get Started

You may not realize it, but you're in a pretty powerful place right now. You're motivated. You're brimming over with self-awareness. You've set a personalized weight loss goal. You've set an activity goal. You know how to pick and prepare good-tasting, good-for-you foods. And, we are standing right here beside you, ready to help you every step of the way.

Smart Start is the 28-day beginning of *Get Skinny the Smart Way*. We have set up 28 days of menus for you to eat and enjoy, guaranteed to help you lose weight quickly. **Smart Start** jump starts your weight loss. By the end of the month you'll be thinner and more physically fit, and ready to move on to the next phase, **Moving Along**, in Chapter 10.

You'll see that we plan all meals and snacks for the first 14 days. During the second 14 days of **Smart Start**, we turn over some of that responsibility to you. Our ultimate goal is to put you in control. Some of our clients feel they aren't ready for that step so soon. Some of them like to cycle through **Smart Start** two or three times or they prefer to cycle through the first 14 days a second time and then move on, stretching **Smart Start** into a 6 week plan. That's okay, too. We have confidence you will pick the approach that is best for you. As we've told you many times before, the beauty of *Your Personalized Weight Attack Plan* is that it can be personalized for you.

3 Meals + 3 Snacks

Eat regular meals plus a snack or two is a thin habit. Small frequent meals lead to more satisfaction and less overeating. The key is planning and we've done that for you. Planning meals and snacks prevents spontaneous eating. It can also reduce your anxiety about eating because you know what the day will hold.

Smart Start menus contain 3 meals and 3 snacks every day. We've done this because many of our clients have had difficulty sticking with their dieting goals if they have to go long stretches without food. As you get more secure taking charge of how you eat, you may find that 1 or 2 snacks are enough each day. But in the meantime, stick with the plan. It works!

Breakfast Counts

Eat breakfast is a thin habit because it's the most important meal of the day. It breaks the overnight fast and revs up your body. Breakfast eaters burn calories more efficiently and are thinner than breakfast skippers.

Many of our clients tell us they aren't hungry in the morning. We believe they need to relearn the feeling of morning hunger because their body needs fuel. As you'll see, the **Smart Start** breakfast choices are varied because breakfast is the meal people vary the least. Most of us find a few things we enjoy and stick with them. For the more adventurous we offer options. If you like some of the choices better than others, repeat the ones you prefer.

Fruits and Veggies

More fruits and vegetables, less juice is a thin habit. Though juices are healthy choices, they are more calorie dense and don't offer the chewing satisfaction of the whole fruit or vegetable. Until you reach your target weight, it is wiser to "chew" than "drink" your fruits and veggies.

Smart Start menus are planned to include 5 fruits and vegetables each day—the experts' recommendation. This not only offers you protection against many serious health problems but is a simple way to lose weight faster. Fruits and vegetables are full of nutrients and low in calories.

Although we've always found it easy to carry and eat fresh fruit, many of our clients don't like to do this. A simple alternative is individual servings of sliced fruit or fruit sauces (a great place to stir in pectin). They come in handy 4- and 6-packs which can be kept in your desk drawer, car or bag. Most supermarkets, delis and even the office coffee cart, now offer cut-up fresh fruit—another option to get your 5 a day.

Potatoes count—and are an easy way to get 1 vegetable a day. And don't forget salads. In Chapter 8 you saw how easy it was to "Build A Better Salad," bursting with color, nutrients, fiber and very few calories. Any other vegetables you enjoy—raw or cooked—are good choices, too. We've planned fruit, salad and vegetable choices for the **Smart Start** menus and if you don't like our choices, pick your own. Just remember, the goal is to eat 5 a day.

Go Easy on Bread and Pasta

We love bread and pasta but we also realize that eating too many servings a day can be a dieter's downfall. So, for the next 28 days, we are going to limit bread and pasta to no more than 4 commonsense servings a day. You'll be getting carbohydrates from many other foods—fruits, vegetables, beans, milk and yogurt. We are not putting you on a low carbohydrate diet. We're just temporarily limiting foods that can stall weight loss.

Get Skinny's Powerful Dieting Aids

Pectin Power

Pectin is a powerful hunger chaser when added to foods. It slows down the emptying of your stomach, making you feel fuller longer. In **Smart Start** we encourage you to include a pectin hunger chaser every day to blunt your appetite and help you lose weight faster.

You'll find that yogurt is a good place to add pectin. It combines nicely with the texture and yogurt is an excellent source of calcium, another powerful dieting aid.

Beside yogurt, pectin can be stirred into soup, hot cereal, mashed potatoes, smoothies, applesauce, fruit sauce, pudding, milk, flavored milk, fruit and vegetable juice. Our clients have been pretty inventive adding pectin to foods. We're sure you'll be, too.

Pectin can be added to any food at any time of the day. We recommend starting with 1 teaspoon and gradually adding more, to a maximum of 1 tablespoon (3 teaspoons) a day. You can divide the pectin into 1, 2 or 3 portions, adding 1 teaspoon to food at varying times throughout the day. Or you can use one portion (1 to 3 teaspoons) added to one food. There may be a time in the day when you are more likely to overeat. To combat this, use pectin then to make you more satisfied with less.

Calcium Counts

We have planned two calcium-rich foods for each **Smart Start** menu. In addition, we recommend a daily calcium supplement of 600 milligrams. This combination will ensure you get 1200 milligrams of calcium each day. Why is this so important? Population surveys have shown that people who get 1100 milligrams of calcium a day had the lowest risk of being overweight. But less than 10% of women and 25% of men get enough calcium daily. And only 25% of women and 14% of men take a daily calcium supplement.

Research done by Dr. Robert Heaney and his colleagues at Creighton University showed that people with the highest calcium intake had the lowest BMIs (Body Mass Index). And adequate calcium can prevent midlife weight gain in women. Calcium helps your body use up fat rather than store it.

If you use yogurt to make your daily hunger chaser, you get a two-for-one dieting aid—pectin to make you feel fuller longer and calcium to use up fat faster. The best sources of calcium are yogurt, milk, cheese, calcium-fortified foods, and supplements. In Chapters 5 and 8 you'll find more information on the benefits of calcium and how to make your eating plan calcium-rich.

SMART STUFF

Nonfat yogurt is the best source of calcium in the American diet, followed by milk. Calcium-fortified soy milk is the best nondairy source.

Water Works

It sounds a little odd, that water with no calories helps you burn calories. But that's exactly what happens. When you don't drink enough water you burn fewer calories. It's been estimated that 75% of Americans regularly drink too little water. Even mild dehydration slows down your metabolism by 3%, which for the average person can add up to almost 20,000 unused calories in a year.

From now on we want you to drink at least 8 glasses of water or other fluids each day. Juice, soup, milk, herbal teas and decaffeinated soda, tea and coffee count just like water. Count only half of the caffeine-containing soda, tea and coffee you drink. And don't count any alcohol toward you daily water goal. Both caffeine and alcohol dehydrate you but alcohol is a more powerful water waster.

SMART STUFF—Color counts

The color of your urine is a simple way to tell if you are drinking enough fluids. The deeper the yellow the more likely you are mildly dehydrated. Pale yellow to clear means good hydration.

Keeping Track

Calories

Your Target Calorie Zone is: ____ calories per day.

Write it down and you'll lose. Studies have shown that keeping a daily food diary is a powerful ally when losing weight. Just keeping track of what you eat is guaranteed to cut calorie intake by 10% a day. That's more than 100 calories lost a day.

We know that keeping a food diary works, but many of our clients resist doing it. Therefore, we've learned to compromise. We suggest that you keep a food diary, daily, for the first 7 days on **Smart Start**. After that, record everything you eat for 2 or 3 days each week as a check to be sure you are still on target. We also recommend using the daily food diary during stressful times— changing jobs, holidays, vacations—any situation that might derail you from your goals.

You may be wondering why it's important to keep a food diary if the **Smart Start** menus are already planned. Your Daily Food Diary makes sure you stay within your target calorie zone.

Women, who typically are smaller and need less calories than men, may need to choose the less calorie dense choices from each commonsense portion category. A snack-size yogurt, for your A.M. snack, is an example of how to get what you need on a smaller scale. Add-ons also add up, so you'll want to note those toppings we often add without thinking.

And we realize that you might make your own personal adjustments to the menus we've planned because of likes, dislikes and availability. In this way keeping track keeps you on target.

In Appendix 3, there is a Daily Food Diary form and instructions on the best way to use it to your advantage.

SMART STUFF

Most of us enjoy a drink—a beer or a glass of wine. An occasional drink will not sabotage your dieting goals. There's even evidence to suggest that moderate drinking has health benefits. But all alcoholic drinks have calories and research shows that most people underreport what they drink.

Activity

Your Weekly Activity Goal is: ____ calories burned through activity.

Move it and lose it. Activity revs up your body's metabolism so you use more calories and burn them faster. A diet without exercise won't work in the long run. That's why the *Get Skinny* diet builds in activity right from the start. In Chapter 7 you set your own individualized activity goal. You'll modify this goal as your fitness level goes up and your weight comes down.

Everything counts, from everyday activities like gardening and shoveling snow, to social activities like dancing and a round of golf, to structured exercise programs like martial arts, spinning or step aerobic classes. Any activity you do for 10 minutes or more counts toward your weekly activity goal. As with everything else on the *Get Skinny* diet, you'll personalize your activity plan by picking the activities you most enjoy. It doesn't matter what you do, it's just important that you do it regularly.

SMART STUFF

Forty-one percent of overweight women and 37% of overweight men don't do any regular physical activity.

—Centers for Disease Control and Prevention

In Chapter 6 there's more information on everyday activities that count toward your activity goal, as well as information on walking—an all-time great calorie burner—along with the benefits of strength training and stretching. In Appendix 2 there is a basic strength training and stretching program. In Appendix 1, there is a Weekly Activity Log form and instructions on the best way to use it to your advantage.

Smart Start Menus

Each **Smart Start** menu gives food choices for breakfast, A.M. snack, lunch, afternoon snack, dinner and P.M. snack, along with the commonsense portion for each food. Depending on your individual target calorie zone, you may be able to eat more than one commonsense portion.

GET SKINNY AT A GLANCE

It's hard to remember everything about eating well and being active, so here is a quick reference when you need a refresher. To learn more about:

You may also substitute foods for those we recommend. When you do this, stick with commonsense portion sizes and track the calories of your choice.

Always include beverages with meals. Water is our first choice, followed by flavored seltzer, green tea, herbal tea, diet iced tea, diet lemonade and diet soda, all of which are calorie free. Nonfat milk is a good-tasting, low calorie, calcium-rich choice, as well. A few cups of coffee or tea are fine; just remember only half of these drinks count toward your 8 cups of water a day. Select your favorites.

Throughout the menus, you'll see that we've given you tips, recipes and even some nutrition information to help you eat smart.

* = Smart Tip

R = Smart Recipe

Smart Start Menus

Week 1 and 2
Day 1 to 14

We've set up 14 days of menus with a wide variety of foods. They'll offer you an opportunity to try some new taste combinations and some new foods. Exploring new options should be part of *Your Personalized Weight Attack Plan.*

If there is any food or meal that is not to your taste, just substitute another choice. To encourage you to have a cup of fat-burning green tea, we've included a cup almost every day for breakfast. If you'd prefer your usual morning cup of coffee, have a cup of green tea for a "coffee break" at work or sip a cup while relaxing in the evening.

For the first week of **Smart Start**, keep track of calories every day on your Daily Food Diary (page 330). During the second week of **Smart Start**, track calories for 2 to 3 days during the week to be sure you're on target with your calorie zone.

And remember, keep track of your daily activities on your Weekly Activity Log (page 298).

Smart Start Menu

Day 1

Breakfast	**Commonsense Serving**
Ready-to-eat cereal +	1 cup
nonfat milk	1 cup
Banana	1 medium
Whole wheat toast +	1 slice
all fruit jelly★	1 tablespoon
Green tea★	

A.M. Snack

Nonfat yogurt + pectin	8-ounce container★

Lunch

Roast beef chef's salad★	
Salad	2 cups
Thin sliced deli roast beef	2 ounces
Reduced-calorie salad	2 tablespoons
dressing	
Whole wheat crackers	5
Diet lemonade	

Afternoon Snack

Apple	1 medium

Dinner

Mustard Chicken Breasts[R]	4 ounces
Baked potato	1 medium
Steamed asparagus	1 cup
Flavored seltzer	

P.M. Snack

Popcorn	2 cups

Smart Start Menu

Day 1

*Smart Tip: All fruit spreads have fewer calories per tablespoon than regular jam or jelly. Jam or jelly has fewer calories per tablespoon than margarine or butter.

*Smart Tip: A cup of green tea a day helps you burn fat faster.

*Smart Tip: Women may find that a 4-ounce, snack-size nonfat yogurt will be more than enough for their A.M. snack.

*Smart Tip: Prewashed bagged salads come in unending varieties, making it easy to prepare tasty salads in no time. Keep a couple of different choices on hand.

[R]**Smart Recipe**
Mustard Chicken Breasts, page 149

Smart Start Menu

Day 2

Breakfast	**Commonsense Serving**
Oatmeal* +	1 cup
nonfat milk	1 cup
Blueberries	1 cup
Green tea	

A.M. Snack

Nonfat yogurt + pectin	8-ounce container*

Lunch

Open-face swiss and tomato	1 slice whole wheat bread
sandwich	1 slice swiss cheese
	2 slices tomato
	1 teaspoon reduced-calorie italian dressing
Fresh cucumber spears	1 cup
Diet soda	

Afternoon Snack

Orange	1 medium

Dinner

Soy* (garden) burger with salsa	3–4 ounces
on whole wheat roll	1
Golden Onions & Mushrooms^R	1 cup
Tossed salad	2 cups
Reduced-calorie salad dressing	2 tablespoons
Flavored seltzer	

P.M. Snack

Sorbet	½ cup

Smart Start Menu
Day 2

*Smart Tip: If you are too rushed in the morning to have breakfast at home, keep packets of oatmeal in your desk drawer to make in the office microwave.

*Smart Tip: Women may find a 4-ounce, snack-size nonfat yogurt will be more than enough for their A.M. snack.

*Smart Tip: Frozen and refrigerated soy (garden) burgers are available in many flavors, they are moderate in calories, low in fat, rich in fiber and as rich in protein as meat.

RSmart Recipe

Golden Brown Onions & Mushrooms

2 large onions, sliced
1 cup sliced mushrooms (6–8)
2 teaspoons teriyaki sauce

Spray a frying pan with nonstick cooking spray. Fry onions and mushrooms on medium-high heat, 5 to 7 minutes until soft and brown. Stir in teriyaki sauce and serve.

Serving size = 1 cup   40 calories

Smart Start Menu

Day 3

Breakfast	Commonsense Serving
Toasted mini bagels +	2
light cream cheese	2 tablespoons
Grapefruit	½
Green tea★	

A.M. Snack

Nonfat yogurt + pectin	8-ounce container★

Lunch

Pita pocket stuffed with	1 small
Mediterranean Bulgur Salad^R	1 cup
Red pepper strips	1 cup
Nonfat milk★	1 cup

Afternoon Snack

Pear	1 medium

Dinner

Horseradish Crusted Flounder^R	4 ounces
Microwave Tomatoes^R	1 cup
Brown rice	1 cup
Flavored seltzer★	

P.M. Snack

Glass of red wine	4 ounces

Smart Start Menu

Day 3

★Smart Tip: Mix and match the beverages of your choice throughout the day. Our suggestions will help you remember to:
- Have 8 glasses of water or other fluids a day
- Drink at least 1 glass of nonfat milk a day to be sure you get enough calcium
- Enjoy a cup of fat-burning green tea daily.

★Smart Tip: Women may find a 4-ounce, snack-size nonfat yogurt will be more than enough for their A.M. snack.

ᴿSmart Recipe
Mediterranean Bulgur Salad, page 138
Microwave Tomatoes, page 153

Horseradish Crusted Flounder

1 pound flounder fillets
3 tablespoons horseradish
3 tablespoons nonfat plain yogurt
3 tablespoons seasoned breadcrumbs

Preheat broiler. Spray a baking pan with nonfat cooking spray, place fillets on pan. Mix together horseradish, breadcrumbs and yogurt; spread mixture on fish. Broil 5 minutes until fish flakes. Makes 4 servings.

1 serving = 4 ounces   180 calories

Smart Start Menu

Day 4

Breakfast	**Commonsense Serving**
Breakfast burrito	
Scrambled egg	1
Wrap	1, 6-inch
Salsa	
Sliced strawberries	1 cup
Green tea	

A.M. Snack

Nonfat yogurt + pectin	8-ounce container★

Lunch

High Energy Drink[R]	1 serving

Afternoon Snack

Peach	1 medium

Dinner

Oven Roasted Pork Tenderloin[R]	4 ounces
Oven Roasted Seasoned Red Potatoes★[R]	1 cup
Applesauce	½ cup
Steamed broccoli	1 cup
Herbal tea	

P.M. Snack

Nonfat ready-to-eat vanilla pudding	½ cup

Smart Start Menu

Day 4

Smart Tip: Women may find a 4-ounce, snack-size nonfat yogurt will be more than enough for their A.M. snack.

Smart Tip: Eating the skins on red potatoes adds some extra fiber at dinner.

RSmart Recipe

High Energy Drink, page 144

Oven Roasted Pork Tenderloin, page 147

Oven Roasted Seasoned Red Potatoes

Paprika

Lemon pepper

Garlic powder

12 small red potatoes, scrubbed and halved

Coat a baking dish with nonfat cooking spray. Generously sprinkle the surface of the dish with paprika, lemon pepper and garlic powder. Place potatoes on baking dish, cut side down. Lightly spray potatoes with nonfat cooking spray. Sprinkle potatoes with spices. Bake at 425° F for 30 minutes.

1 cup = 1 serving   150 calories

Smart Start Menu

Day 5

Breakfast	**Commonsense Serving**
Toaster waffles +	2
honey*	2 teaspoons
Sliced papaya	1 cup
Green tea	

A.M. Snack

Nonfat yogurt + pectin	8-ounce container*

Lunch

Sliced egg sandwich with	2 slices whole wheat bread
romaine lettuce and salsa	1 sliced egg
Celery sticks	1 cup
Diet iced tea	

Afternoon Snack

Grapes	1 cup

Dinner

Tangy Cottage Cheese Fruit Salad^R	1 salad
Whole wheat dinner roll	1
Flavored seltzer	

P.M. Snack

Fudgesicle	1

Smart Start Menu
Day 5

★Smart Tip: Honey has less calories (42 in 2 tsp.) than pancake syrup (57 in 1 tbsp.) or try light pancake syrup or all fruit jelly.

★Smart Tip: Women may find a 4-ounce, snack-size nonfat yogurt will be more than enough for their A.M. snack.

ᴿSmart Recipe

Tangy Cottage Cheese Salad

2 cups salad greens
½ cup nonfat cottage cheese
¼ cup mandarin orange sections
1 apple, thinly sliced
½ cup blueberries
2 tablespoons, thinly sliced red onion

Place salad greens on a plate. Place cottage cheese in the center and arrange fruit around plate. Scatter onion rings on top of salad.

1 serving = 1 salad   346 calories

Smart Start Menu
Day 6

Breakfast	**Commonsense Serving**
Fruit Smoothie[R]	1 serving

A.M. Snack

Nonfat yogurt + pectin	8-ounce container*

Lunch

Tuna niçoise salad

Salad	2 cups
Tuna in water	2 ounces (¼ cup)
Anchovy fillets	2
Reduced-calorie thousand island dressing	2 tablespoons
Green tea	

Afternoon Snack

Fresh watermelon chunks	1 cup

Dinner

Slow-Cooked Hawaiian Chicken[R]	4 ounces
Brown rice	1 cup
Steamed green beans	1 cup
Flavored seltzer	

P.M. Snack

Chocolate Slush[R]	1 serving

Smart Start Menu

Day 6

Smart Tip: Women may find a 4-ounce, snack-size nonfat yogurt will be more than enough for their A.M. snack.

[R]**Smart Recipes**
Fruit Smoothie, page 143

Slow-Cooked Hawaiian Chicken

With a slow cooker you can put this dish together in minutes in the morning and come home to a hot meal at night. Chicken thighs and legs are better for long cooking.

1½ pounds skinless chicken legs and thighs
1 can (8 ounces) crushed pineapple
3 tablespoons cider vinegar
3 tablespoons teriyaki sauce
1 tablespoon grated fresh ginger or ½ teaspoon dried

Spray an electric slow cooker with nonstick cooking spray. Put chicken in slow cooker and add remaining ingredients. Cook on low 8 hours.

Makes 6 servings.   1 serving = 240 calories

Chocolate Slush

Combine 1 cup nonfat milk, 2 tablespoons chocolate syrup and 6 ice cubes in a blender container and process until slushy, about 30 seconds.

1 single serving   180 calories

Smart Start Menu

Day 7

Breakfast	**Commonsense Serving**
Lowfat corned beef hash	½ cup
Whole wheat toast★ +	1 slice
all fruit jelly	1 tablespoon
Orange sections	1 cup
Green tea	

A.M. Snack

Nonfat yogurt + pectin	8-ounce container★

Lunch

Pita pocket stuffed with salad +	1 small pita + 1 cup salad
shredded cheese and	2 tablespoons
reduced-calorie salad dressing	1 tablespoon
Dill pickle	1 large
Nonfat milk	1 cup

Afternoon Snack

Tangerines	2

Dinner

Broiled flank steak	4 ounces
Confetti Couscous^R	1 cup
Tossed salad +	2 cups
reduced-calorie salad dressing	2 tablespoons
Flavored seltzer	

P.M. Snack

Pretzel sticks	30 (1 ounce)

Smart Start Menu

Day 7

⋆**Smart Tip:** Vary bread choices by trying other fiber-rich varieties—oatmeal, multigrain or rye.

⋆**Smart Tip:** Women may find a 4-ounce, snack-size nonfat yogurt will be more than enough for their A.M. snack.

[R]**Smart Recipe**
Confetti Couscous, page 138

Smart Start Menu

Day 8

Breakfast	**Commonsense Serving**
Ready-to-eat cereal +	1 cup
nonfat milk	1 cup
Banana	1 medium
Whole wheat toast +	1 slice
all fruit jelly	1 tablespoon
Green tea	

A.M. Snack	
Nonfat yogurt + pectin	8-ounce container★

Lunch	
Roast beef wrap with	1, 6-inch
coleslaw +	2 ounces deli roast beef
reduced-calorie creamy	½ cup coleslaw mix
salad dressing	1 tablespoon
Raw baby carrots	1 cup
Diet soda	

Afternoon Snack	
Fresh pineapple chunks	1 cup

Dinner	
Ginger Tofu^R	1 cup
Brown rice	1 cup
Steamed pea pods	1 cup
Flavored seltzer	

P.M. Snack	
Vanilla frozen yogurt★	½ cup

Smart Start Menu

Day 8

★Smart Tip: Women may find a 4-ounce, snack-size nonfat yogurt will be more than enough for their A.M. snack.

★Smart Tip: Many brands of frozen yogurt have more calcium in a serving than reduced-calorie ice cream.

ᴿSmart Recipe
Ginger Tofu, page 154

Smart Start Menu

Day 9

Breakfast	**Commonsense Serving**
Oatmeal★ +	1 cup
nonfat milk	1 cup
Honeydew	⅒ melon
Green tea	

A.M. Snack

Nonfat yogurt + pectin	8-ounce container★

Lunch

Sliced egg chef's salad +	2 cups salad
	1 hard-cooked sliced egg
reduced-calorie salad dressing	2 tablespoons
Breadsticks	2
Herbal tea	

Afternoon Snack

Kiwis	2

Dinner

Lemon Fish Steaks^R	4 ounces
Kasha Delight^R	1 cup
Steamed broccoli	1 cup
Flavored seltzer	

P.M. Snack

Popcorn	2 cups

Smart Start Menu

Day 9

*Smart Tip:** To make a richer tasting, calcium-rich oatmeal, substitute nonfat milk for water when cooking or heating in the microwave.

*Smart Tip:** Women may find a 4-ounce, snack-size nonfat yogurt will be more than enough for their A.M. snack.

---

^R**Smart Recipes**
Lemon Fish Steaks, page 148
Kasha Delight, page 138

Smart Start Menu

Day 10

Breakfast	Commonsense Serving
Toasted English muffin +	1
all fruit jelly	1 tablespoon
Fresh strawberries	1 cup
Green tea	

A.M. Snack	
Nonfat yogurt + pectin	8-ounce container*

Lunch	
Ham sandwich	2 ounces deli ham
	2 slices whole wheat bread
	Lettuce
	Mustard*
Dill pickle	1 large pickle
Diet soda	

Afternoon Snack	
Plum	2 small or 1 medium

Dinner	
Southwestern Chili Stew with	1 cup
Polenta^R	2 slices
Fresh cucumber spears	1 cup
Nonfat milk	1 cup

P.M. Snack	
Lemon Ice^R	½ cup

Smart Start Menu

Day 10

***Smart Tip:** Women may find a 4-ounce, snack-size nonfat yogurt will be more than enough for their A.M. snack.

***Smart Tip:** Mustard and horseradish prevent bacteria from growing, keeping your sandwich safe from spoiling.

---

^RSmart Recipe

Lemon Ice, page 154

Southwestern Chili Stew with Polenta

1 large pepper (green, yellow or red), seeded and chopped or
   1 cup frozen sliced peppers
2 cups frozen or 1 can (15 ounces) corn
1 can (15 oz) black beans, drained and rinsed well
1 can (14 oz) chili-flavored diced tomatoes
1 cup water
1 teaspoon chili powder or more to taste
1 teaspoon ground cumin
1 tube (1 pound) ready-to-heat polenta

Spray a heavy pot with nonstick cooking spray. Fry pepper for 5 minutes. Stir in remaining ingredients and bring to a boil; reduce heat to simmer and cook uncovered for 20 minutes, stirring occasionally. Slice polenta into ½-inch slices and place on a microwave safe pan; heat on high 2 minutes. Place 2 slices of polenta on a plate, top with 1 cup of stew.

Serving size = 2 slices of polenta + 1 cup stew
192 calories per serving

Smart Start Menu

Day 11

Breakfast	Commonsense Serving
Toasted mini bagels +	2
light cream cheese	2 tablespoons
Cantaloupe	¼ melon
Green tea	

A.M. Snack	
Nonfat yogurt + pectin	8-ounce container*

Lunch	
High Energy Drink[R]	1 serving

Afternoon Snack	
Apricots	3 small

Dinner	
Worcestershire Medley Pasta Sauce[R]	1 cup
Cooked ziti	2 cups
Tossed salad +	2 cups
reduced-calorie dressing	2 tablespoons
Flavored seltzer	

P.M. Snack	
Glass of red wine*	4 ounces

Smart Start Menu

Day 11

★**Smart Tip:** Women may find a 4-ounce, snack-size nonfat yogurt will be more than enough for their A.M. snack.

★**Smart Tip:** Red wines have higher levels of *resveratrol,* a naturally occurring substance found in grapes that reduces the risk of heart disease and cancer.

ᴿSmart Recipes

High Energy Drink, page 144

Worcestershire Medley Pasta Sauce, page 155

Smart Start Menu
Day 12

Breakfast	**Commonsense Serving**
Breakfast burrito	
Scrambled egg	1
Wrap	1, 6-inch
Salsa	
Sliced strawberries	1 cup
Nonfat milk	1 cup

A.M. Snack

Nonfat yogurt + pectin	8-ounce container*

Lunch

Roasted chicken chef's salad	2 ounces sliced ready-to-eat chicken
	2 cups salad
with reduced-calorie salad dressing	2 tablespoons
Saltines	6
Diet iced tea	

Afternoon Snack

Snack-pack applesauce	1 snack pack (4 ounces)

Dinner

Oven Roasted Beef Tenderloin[R]	4 ounces
Baked potato*	1 medium
Roasted Italian Zucchini Slices[R]	3 to 4 slices
Green tea	

P.M. Snack

Pineapple Slush Cocktail[R]	1 serving

Smart Start Menu

Day 12

*__Smart Tip:__ Women may find a 4-ounce, snack-size nonfat yogurt will be more than enough for their A.M. snack.

*__Smart Tip:__ A medium baked potato contains nearly half of your daily vitamin C requirement and is an excellent source of potassium, fiber and disease-fighting antioxidants.

__RSmart Recipes__
Oven Roasted Beef Tenderloin, page 147
Pineapple Slush Cocktail, page 144

Roasted Italian Zucchini Slices

2 medium (6-inch) zucchinis
Italian salad dressing mix

Coat a baking dish with nonfat cooking spray. Wash zucchini; trim off stem end and cut lengthwise into 3 or 4 (¼-inch thick) slices. Place zucchini on baking dish and spray slices lightly with nonfat cooking spray. Sprinkle slices with salad dressing mix. Bake at 400° F for 15 minutes.

1 serving = 3 to 4 slices   28 calories

Smart Start Menu
Day 13

Breakfast	**Commonsense Serving**
Fruit Smoothie[R]	1 serving

A.M. Snack
Nonfat yogurt + pectin	8-ounce container*

Lunch
Refried Bean Wrap[R]	2
Tangy Tomato Salad[R]	1 cup
Diet iced tea	

Afternoon Snack
Fresh mixed fruit salad	1 cup

Dinner
Baked lean ham	4 ounces
Baked sweet potato*	1 medium
Steamed asparagus spears	1 cup
Whole wheat dinner roll	1
Flavored seltzer	

P.M. Snack
Animal crackers	10
Green tea	1 cup

Smart Start Menu

Day 13

*Smart Tip: Women may find a 4-ounce, snack-size nonfat yogurt will be more than enough for their A.M. snack.

*Smart Tip: Sweet potatoes are such an excellent source of vitamin A that one serving has almost 5 times the daily recommended amount.

ᴿSmart Recipes
Fruit Smoothie, page 143

Refried Bean Wrap

Spread 1 (6-inch) wrap with ¼ cup nonfat refried beans, top with 1 tablespoon nonfat sour cream, 2 tablespoons chopped cucumber, 2 tablespoons chopped red pepper and ½ cup shredded lettuce.

1 wrap   185 calories

Tangy Tomato Salad

2 large tomatoes, sliced
1 small onion, sliced
1 tablespoon fresh parsley
2 tablespoons nonfat raspberry vinaigrette

Beginning with tomatoes, layer tomato slices, onion and parsley in a small dish; drizzle with dressing. Best served at room temperature.

Serving size = 1 cup   49 calories

Smart Start Menu
Day 14

Breakfast	**Commonsense Serving**
Toaster waffles +	2
honey	2 teaspoons
Sliced mango	1 cup
Green tea	

A.M. Snack

Nonfat yogurt + pectin	8-ounce container*

Lunch

Sliced egg sandwich with	2 slices whole wheat
romaine lettuce and salsa	bread
	1 sliced egg
Cherry tomatoes	1 cup
Mineral water	1 cup

Afternoon Snack

Snack-pack sliced peaches in	1 snack pack (4 ounces)
light syrup	

Dinner

Scallops in Wine Sauce^R	1 serving
Thin spaghetti	2 cups
Steamed spinach*	1 cup
Flavored seltzer	

P.M. Snack

Light hot chocolate*	1 cup

Smart Start Menu

Day 14

*Smart Tip: Women may find a 4-ounce, snack-size nonfat yogurt will be more than enough for their A.M. snack.

*Smart Tip: Spinach has more antioxidants in a serving than any other vegetable but kale, protecting you against diseases and the effects of aging.

*Smart Tip: Making hot chocolate with nonfat milk instead of water is an added calcium boost.

R Smart Recipe

Scallops in Wine Sauce

2 cloves garlic, minced
1 pound bay or sea scallops
12 cherry tomatoes, cut in half
⅓ cup dry white wine (regular or nonalcoholic)
1 tablespoon fresh parsley or 1 teaspoon dried

Coat a frying pan with nonstick cooking spray, fry garlic for 1 minute until soft; add scallops, tomatoes and wine. Cook 4 to 5 minutes until scallops have turned white. Sprinkle with parsley to serve.

Makes 4 servings   1 serving = 126 calories

Smart Start Menus

Week 3
Day 15 to 21

As we've said from the beginning, our goal is to put you in control. So, for the next week, you'll be planning lunch. You can either pick your favorites from Week 1 and 2 or plan anything you like. Just stick with commonsense portions and keep track of the calories to stay within your target calorie zone.

We'd recommend using your Daily Food Diary (page 330) 2 or 3 times during the week to be sure you stay on target.

Keep track of your daily activities using your Weekly Activity Log (page 298).

Smart Start Menu

Day 15

Breakfast	**Commonsense Serving**
Breakfast burrito	
Scrambled egg	1
Wrap	1, 6-inch
Salsa	
Red grapefruit sections	1 cup
Green tea	

A.M. Snack

Nonfat yogurt + pectin	8-ounce container★

Lunch★

_____   _____
_____   _____
_____   _____
_____   _____

Afternoon Snack

Banana	1 medium

Dinner

Roasted turkey breast	4 ounces
Quick-Baked Acorn Squash^R	1 cup
Steamed green beans	1 cup
Wholeberry cranberry sauce★	2 tablespoons
Flavored seltzer	

P.M. Snack

Italian ice cup	1

Smart Start Menu

Day 15

*Smart Tip: Women may find a 4-ounce, snack-size nonfat yogurt will be more than enough for their A.M. snack.

*Smart Tip: Remember to have a second calcium-rich food today.

*Smart Tip: Wholeberry cranberries have more fiber than jellied cranberries.

R Smart Recipe

Quick-Baked Acorn Squash

Wash, cut in half and seed a ¾ pound acorn squash. Lightly coat a microwave-safe pan with nonfat cooking spray. Place squash cut side down on pan and microwave on high for 10 minutes. Turn squash over and add 2 teaspoons brown sugar to each half. Continue cooking 5 minutes or until squash is fork tender.

1 serving = ½ squash   120 calories

Smart Start Menu

Day 16

Breakfast	Commonsense Serving
Ready-to-eat cereal +	1 cup
nonfat milk	1 cup
Fresh raspberries★	1 cup
Whole wheat toast +	1 slice
all fruit jelly	1 tablespoon
Green tea	

A.M. Snack

Nonfat yogurt + pectin	8-ounce container★

Lunch

_____	_____
_____	_____
_____	_____
_____	_____

Afternoon Snack

Mandarin orange sections	½ cup

Dinner

Reduced-calorie beef	1
or poultry hot dog +	
roll★	1
Sauerkraut	1 cup
Vegetarian baked beans	½ cup
Flavored seltzer	

P.M. Snack

Ready-to-eat nonfat chocolate	½ cup
pudding	

Smart Start Menu

Day 16

★Smart Tip: Blueberries, raspberries and strawberries are excellent sources of health-protecting antioxidants.

★Smart Tip: Women may find a 4-ounce, snack-size nonfat yogurt will be more than enough for their A.M. snack.

★Smart Tip: Use whole wheat or multigrain hot dog rolls for added fiber.

Smart Start Menu

Day 17

Breakfast	**Commonsense Serving**
Oatmeal +	1 cup
nonfat milk	1 cup
Cantaloupe	¼ melon
Green tea	

A.M. Snack

Nonfat yogurt + pectin	8-ounce container★

Lunch

_____   _____

_____   _____

_____   _____

_____   _____

Afternoon Snack

Apple	1 medium

Dinner	
Spicy Fish[R]	4 ounces
Brown rice★	1 cup
Steamed baby carrots	1 cup
Flavored seltzer	

P.M. Snack

Fruit sorbet	½ cup

Smart Start Menu

Day 17

*Smart Tip: Women may find a 4-ounce, snack-size nonfat yogurt will be more than enough for their A.M. snack.

*Smart Tip: A simple trick to add flavor without calories is to lightly spray rice with a flavored cooking spray—lemon, butter, garlic, or olive oil—and top with a sprinkle of fresh pepper.

RSmart Recipe
Spicy Fish, page 148

Smart Start Menu

Day 18

Breakfast	**Commonsense Serving**
Breakfast cheese danish	
Toasted whole wheat	1
English muffin	
Nonfat ricotta cheese	¼ cup
Cinnamon sugar	¼ teaspoon
Fresh strawberries	1 cup
Green tea	

A.M. Snack

Nonfat yogurt + pectin	8-ounce container★

Lunch

_____   _____

_____   _____

_____   _____

_____   _____

Afternoon Snack

Orange	1 medium

Dinner

Barbecue Chicken Sandwich^R	1 sandwich
Balsamic Cucumber Salad^R	1 cup
Flavored seltzer	

P.M. Snack

Fudgesicle	1

Smart Start Menu

Day 18

*Smart Tip: Women may find a 4–ounce, snack–size nonfat yogurt will be more than enough for their A.M. snack.

^R**Smart Recipes**
Balsamic Cucumber Salad, page 153

Barbecue Chicken Sandwich

½ cup ketchup
2 tablespoons molasses
2 tablespoons cider vinegar
1 tablespoon mustard
4 whole wheat hamburger buns
1 package (10 ounces) ready-to-eat chicken slices
1 cup ready-to-use coleslaw mix (without dressing)

In a microwave–safe bowl, combine ketchup, molasses, vinegar and mustard; stir. Cover to reduce spattering and heat on high 2 to 3 minutes. Divide the chicken between four buns; top each with hot barbecue sauce and ¼ cup coleslaw mix.

1 serving = 1 sandwich   267 calories

Smart Start Menu

Day 19

Breakfast	**Commonsense Serving**
High Energy Drink[R]	1 serving

A.M. Snack
Nonfat yogurt + pectin — 8-ounce container*

Lunch*

_____   _____

_____   _____

_____   _____

_____   _____

Afternoon Snack
Nectarine — 1 medium

Dinner

Smothered Sausage & Onions[R]	1 cup
Bowtie pasta	2 cups
Salad +	2 cups
reduced-fat italian dressing	2 tablespoons

P.M. Snack

Graham crackers	2 squares
Green tea	

Smart Start Menu

Day 19

***Smart Tip:** Women may find a 4-ounce, snack-size nonfat yogurt will be more than enough for their A.M. snack.

***Smart Tip:** Buy calcium-fortified soy milk for the health benefits of soy plus the fat burning benefits of calcium.

[R]**Smart Recipes**

High Energy Drink, page 144

Smothered Sausage & Onions, page 149

Smart Start Menu
Day 20

Breakfast	Commonsense Serving
Toasted mini bagels +	2
light cream cheese	2 tablespoons
Sliced papaya	1 cup
Green tea	

A.M. Snack

Nonfat yogurt + pectin	8-ounce container★

Lunch

_____   _____
_____   _____
_____   _____
_____   _____

Afternoon Snack

Pear	1 medium

Dinner

London broil	4 ounces
Baked potato★	1 medium
Steamed broccoli	1 cup
Flavored seltzer	

P.M. Snack

Glass of red wine★	4 ounces

Smart Start Menu

Day 20

★Smart Tip: Women may find a 4-ounce, snack-size nonfat yogurt will be more than enough for their A.M. snack.

★Smart Tip: Fresh chives, nonfat yogurt, cracked pepper, and butter buds add taste to a baked potato with little or no calories.

★Smart Tip: Add seltzer, ice and a twist of lemon to a glass of wine for a tall refreshing drink on a hot night.

Smart Start Menu

Day 21

Breakfast	**Commonsense Serving**
Raisin bread toasted	1 slice
Nonfat cottage cheese	½ cup
Mixed fruit salad	1 cup
Green tea	

A.M. Snack

Nonfat yogurt + pectin	8-ounce container★

Lunch

_____	_____
_____	_____
_____	_____
_____	_____

Afternoon Snack

Peach	1 medium

Dinner	
Turkey burger★ on a	(3 to 4 ounces)
whole wheat roll topped with	1 roll
shredded lettuce and salsa★	
Greek Cucumber Salad^R	1 cup
Flavored seltzer	

P.M. Snack

Chocolate frozen yogurt	½ cup

Smart Start Menu

Day 21

*Smart Tip: Women may find a 4-ounce, snack-size nonfat yogurt will be more than enough for their A.M. snack.

*Smart Tip: Frozen, seasoned turkey burgers are pre-portioned in commonsense sizes, lower in fat than traditional hamburgers and cook quickly.

*Smart Tip: Salsa comes in numerous flavors—tomato, bean, corn, roasted pepper, artichoke, peach—with degrees of heat from very mild to volcanic, and adds so few calories to a sandwich, you don't even have to count them.

RSmart Recipe

Greek Cucumber Salad

2 large cucumbers
1 cup nonfat plain yogurt
¼ cup loosely packed, chopped fresh mint or 1 tablespoon
   dried
2 cloves garlic, minced
Salt and pepper to taste

Peel cucumbers; cut in half lengthwise and scoop out seeds with a spoon. Slice thinly. Combine remaining ingredients; pour over cucumbers and stir to coat well.

1 serving = 1 cup   72 calories

Smart Start Menus

Week 4

Day 22 to 28

By this point, you should be almost ready to take over. You're losing weight and you're in a daily exercise groove. It's time to take charge of what you'd like to eat.

For Week 4 of **Smart Start**, you'll be planning both lunch and dinner. You can pick your favorites from the earlier weeks or plan anything you'd like. Just stick with commonsense portions and keep track of calories to stay within your target calorie zone.

We'd recommend using your Daily Food Diary (page 330) 2 to 3 times during the week to be sure you stay on target.

Keep track of your daily activities using your Weekly Activity Log (page 298).

Smart Start Menu
Day 22

Breakfast	**Commonsense Serving**
Oatmeal★ +	1 cup
nonfat milk	1 cup
Honeydew melon	⅛ melon
Green tea	

A.M. Snack

Nonfat yogurt + pectin	8-ounce container★

Lunch

_____   _____
_____   _____
_____   _____
_____   _____

Afternoon Snack	
Apple★	1 medium

Dinner

_____   _____
_____   _____
_____   _____
_____   _____

P.M. Snack	
Meringue cookies★	4
Green tea	

Smart Start Menu

Day 22

*Smart Tip: Oatmeal, pectin and apples are all rich in soluble fiber, which helps you lose weight faster and also lowers your cholesterol.

*Smart Tip: Women may find a 4-ounce, snack-size nonfat yogurt will be more than enough for their A.M. snack.

*Smart Tip: Meringues made from egg white and sugar are a low calorie, sweet treat, available in lemon, vanilla and chocolate flavors. Stick with the commonsense portion suggested.

Smart Start Menu
Day 23

Breakfast	**Commonsense Serving**
Ready-to-eat cereal +	1 cup
nonfat milk	1 cup
Banana	1 medium
Whole wheat toast +	1 slice
all fruit jelly	1 tablespoon
Green tea	

A.M. Snack

Nonfat yogurt + pectin	8-ounce container★

Lunch

_____   _____

_____   _____

_____   _____

_____   _____

Afternoon Snack

Grapes	1 cup

Dinner

_____   _____

_____   _____

_____   _____

_____   _____

P.M. Snack

Lemon Ice[R]	1 serving

Smart Start Menu

Day 23

***Smart Tip:** Women may find a 4-ounce, snack-size nonfat yogurt will be more than enough for their A.M. snack.

[R]**Smart Recipe**
Lemon Ice, page 154

Smart Start Menu

Day 24

Breakfast	**Commonsense Serving**
Toaster waffles +	2
honey	2 teaspoons
Raspberries*	1 cup
Green tea	

A.M. Snack

Nonfat yogurt + pectin	8-ounce container*

Lunch

_____	_____
_____	_____
_____	_____
_____	

Afternoon Snack

Plums	2 small or 1 medium

Dinner

_____	_____
_____	_____
_____	_____
_____	_____

P.M. Snack

Vanilla frozen yogurt	½ cup

Smart Start Menu

Day 24

*Smart Tip: Puree raspberries in a blender or food processor, heat 10 seconds in a microwave and use instead of honey or syrup on waffles.

*Smart Tip: Women may find a 4-ounce, snack-size nonfat yogurt will be more than enough for their A.M. snack.

Smart Start Menu

Day 25

Breakfast	**Commonsense Serving**
Breakfast burrito	
Scrambled egg	1
Wrap	1, 6-inch
Salsa	
Sliced mango★	1 cup
Green tea	

A.M. Snack	
Nonfat yogurt + pectin	8-ounce container★

Lunch

_____	_____
_____	_____
_____	_____
_____	_____

Afternoon Snack	
Cherries	1 cup

Dinner

_____	_____
_____	_____
_____	_____
_____	_____

P.M. Snack	
Light hot chocolate	1 cup

Smart Start Menu
Day 25

★Smart Tip: A mango for breakfast gives you almost a full day's supply of vitamin C and almost twice your daily supply of vitamin A.

★Smart Tip: Women may find a 4-ounce, snack-size nonfat yogurt will be more than enough for their A.M. snack.

Smart Start Menu

Day 26

Breakfast	Commonsense Serving
Toasted English muffin +	1
all fruit jelly	1 tablespoon
Glazed Pink Grapefruit[R]	½
Green tea	

A.M. Snack	
Nonfat yogurt + pectin	8-ounce container*

Lunch

_____	_____
_____	_____
_____	_____
_____	_____

Afternoon Snack	
Kiwis	2 small

Dinner

_____	_____
_____	_____
_____	_____
_____	_____

P.M. Snack	
Pineapple Slush Cocktail[R]	1 serving

Smart Start Menu

Day 26

★Smart Tip: Women may find a 4-ounce, snack-size nonfat yogurt will be more than enough for their A.M. snack.

ᴿSmart Recipes
Pineapple Slush Cocktail, page 144

Glazed Pink Grapefruit

Sprinkle 1 teaspoon brown sugar over grapefruit half, microwave on medium 30 seconds.

1 serving = ½ grapefruit   51 calories

Smart Start Menu
Day 27

	Commonsense Serving
Breakfast	
High Energy Drink[R]	1 serving
A.M. Snack	
Nonfat yogurt + pectin	8-ounce container*
Lunch	
_____	_____
_____	_____
_____	_____
_____	_____
Afternoon Snack	
Snack-pack mixed fruit	1 snack pack (4 ounces)
Dinner	
_____	_____
_____	_____
_____	_____
_____	_____
P.M. Snack	
Angelfood cake	1 slice
Green tea	

Smart Start Menu

Day 27

*Smart Tip: Women may find a 4-ounce, snack-size nonfat yogurt will be more than enough for their A.M. snack.

ᴿSmart Recipe
High Energy Drink, page 144

Smart Start Menu

Day 28

Breakfast   **Commonsense Serving**

Breakfast cheese danish
   Toasted raisin bread   1 slice
   Ricotta cheese   ¼ cup
   Cinnamon sugar   ¼ teaspoon
Fresh strawberries   1 cup
Green tea

A.M. Snack

Nonfat yogurt + pectin   8-ounce container★

Lunch

_____   _____
_____   _____
_____   _____
_____   _____

Afternoon Snack

Cut-up watermelon★   1 cup

Dinner

_____   _____
_____   _____
_____   _____
_____   _____

P.M. Snack

Pretzel sticks   30 (1 ounce)

Smart Start Menu

Day 28

★Smart Tip: Women may find a 4-ounce, snack-size nonfat yogurt will be more than enough for their A.M. snack.

★Smart Tip: Watermelon is an excellent source of vitamin C; 1 cup provides 25% of your daily requirement.

Chapter 10

Moving Along— The Road to Success

Everyone resists change, and everyone underestimates their ability to change.

How are you doing? You've been using the **Smart Start** phase of *Get Skinny the Smart Way* for the last 4 to 6 weeks. You've lost weight and you're active most, if not all, days. You should be feeling great. And you should be proud of what you've accomplished.

Now it's time to "move along" to the next phase of *Your Personalized Weight Attack Plan*. It's time to integrate everything you've learned and all your new habits into everyday living while you continue to lose weight.

In **Moving Along** you'll be in charge of planning your menu for the day. Though we encourage you to stick with common-sense portions and use thin habits daily, we know that life throws us a curve ball every now and then. It is those curve balls and unexpected situations that could derail your diet goals and stall your motivation to keep going. We aren't going to let that happen.

Being on a diet is a lot like running a marathon. You see pounds slipping off but you wish you could get to the finish line faster. Runners often talk about hitting a wall. Getting to spots in the race where they find it hard to go on. Dieters hit trouble spots, too. Situations that test their resolve. Times when motivation is low or a week or two where progress is slow, despite all your efforts. There's no question that the road to your target weight will have a few pot holes. But simply anticipating these obstacles and knowing that there is a way around them can guarantee your ultimate success.

Taking Charge in Tough Situations

A large part of how you interact with food has a lot to do with your background and emotions. We can help you modify your eating behaviors that are a result of your life experiences. By adjusting behavior you accomplish two things. First, you put a stop to eating habits that cause you to gain weight. Second, and even more important, you begin to identify your own personal "triggers" to overeating. Once your trouble spots become obvious you can eliminate them or find a way around them.

You think you're unique. You're the only one facing tough situations. Boy, are you wrong! The problems, questions and concerns you have about trying to lose weight are shared by most people. We hear the same questions over and over again. So we thought the easiest way to help you solve your problems is to share the answers to our clients' most frequently asked questions.

Some of our suggestions may seem a little unorthodox. We've learned from working with people that the key to success is flexibility. Not all problems can be solved 100%. But every problem does have a compromise solution, one that will allow you to go forward to reach your target weight.

Oops! What Now?

Often after I eat, and I'm full, I have an overwhelming urge to keep chewing. Why?

Eating is one of our most basic pleasurable experiences. You simply don't want to stop the fun. But you are able to recognize when you're full, which is great. To satisfy the urge to keep chewing, try chewing a piece of gum or sip on a large glass of flavored seltzer or mineral water and chopped ice. Ice is crunchy without calories and cold blunts taste. Both may help you subdue the urge to chew.

Whenever I fight with my husband, I bury my sorrow in a bag of potato chips which destroys all my dieting efforts. Any suggestions?

Fights with people we love are tough to deal with and many times we bury our emotions with food. Though we don't suggest overeating as a response to an emotionally tough time, if you find yourself in that spot, a switch to pretzels or popcorn would be less calorie dense.

If it's too late and you've already eaten the potato chips, let's do some math. A 6-ounce bag of potato chips has 900 calories. To use up the extra calories eaten, we'd suggest cutting 200 calories a day from your eating plan for the next 3 days and adding 10 to 20 minutes extra activity each day. This will compensate for the "oops!"

When I can't sleep, I eat. How do I stop this?

The ideal answer is to tell you not to eat late at night or during the night. In real life, middle of the night noshing is a tough habit to break. This habit is interwoven with an emotional issue you are coping with—a tough boss, difficult teenager, money worries, relationship problems. Separating eating and emotions is hard but it can be done. We're pretty sure that you're not eating because you're hungry. You need to examine what's bothering you and try to work on that issue.

While you are doing that, whenever you are tempted to raid the refrigerator after midnight, think high volume, low calories—popcorn, pretzel sticks, rice cakes, a large noncalorie drink with chopped ice, raw vegetables, a huge hunk of watermelon, a bowl of soup. If ice cream is your midnight munchie of choice, switch to Italian ice or ice pops. Even if you eat more than one, ices are far less calorie dense than ice cream.

Our family is dealing with some serious problems at the moment. How can I stick with my diet plan right now?

Everyone's life gets complicated every now and then. If you wait for life to be calm before you attempt to lose weight, you might be waiting for a long time. Real life is rarely calm!

You can, however, cut yourself some slack. Instead of worrying about losing weight right now, concentrate, instead, on eating well and staying active. You may lose more slowly or you may stay where you are, but you won't backslide by putting on extra pounds.

Sometimes when life is chaotic, a structured eating plan can add some much needed structure to life. Try it.

I have to keep candy and cookies in the house for the kids, that I wind up eating. How can I prevent this?

Don't fool yourself. Are you really buying the candy and cookies for the kids or is it a great excuse to indulge? Buy some treats that are good for the whole family—sorbet, graham crackers, raisin bars. If there are some choices that you are trying to resist, put them out of sight and hopefully out of mind. One of the best gifts you can give your children is to be a good role model. Healthy eating habits are contagious.

What do I do after I've eaten something I shouldn't have, like an unplanned slice of pepperoni pizza?

Resist the "Now I've blown it!" syndrome. There will be days when you eat more than you've planned. There will be times when you can't be active. You will backslide. It's inevitable. Just don't let these glitches derail you. Have a backup plan for such occasions.

You couldn't run today because you had to work overtime. Okay, for the next week, add extra time or distance to your usual workout. Ate that pepperoni slice? Okay, for the next day or two be more choosy with food choices or increase activity to use up those extra calories.

A healthy lifestyle isn't based on one meal or one bout of activity. It's a consistent effort to make good choices and be active, most of the time. When you trip up, just say "Oops!". Forgive yourself and get back on track.

Whenever I go to the bakery I wind up buying and eating something I shouldn't. Sometimes I even eat what I bought on the way home. How do I control this?

Stay out of the bakery. Sounds simple but you may be using those trips as a way to sabotage yourself. Or the bakery may be the place your grandfather took you for a special treat. Self-sabotage happens more often than you may realize. People fear success more than failure. Succeeding at weight loss may be a pretty scary thing. Push that scared feeling aside and stay on track. You deserve to be slimmer and fitter.

If the bakery trip is connected to loving feelings from your past, you need to rescript your memory. The best part of the trip to the bakery, as a child, was the love you felt from your grandfather. The eclair he bought for you didn't love you. Separating food and love is a delicate maneuver.

How can I stop overeating? It makes me feel so guilty.

Guilt is a wasted emotion. It causes you to feel awful about something that has already happened that you can't change. Forget the guilt and concentrate on what is triggering you to overeat.

Are you eating too fast? Your brain needs time to process the fact that you've been fed. In **Smart Start** we encouraged you to try to get in touch with your body's signals for hunger and satisfaction. This takes time. Use the hunger and satisfaction rating scales, on page 173, until you get a clearer signal. Try evaluating your satisfaction mid-meal. This could help short-circuit overeating. Another trick is to create an artificial time-out during mid-meal. Try putting on music and listen to at least one song. Now, reassess your feeling of satisfaction again and then take more to eat if you are not full. Relearning satisfaction or "fullness" is a complex but important lesson.

I eat the most when I'm sad. How can I stop this?

Eating can be comforting. We often reach for food when we feel sad, lonely, frustrated or overwhelmed. Eating pushes the emotion into the background, but not for long. When the feelings return, you eat more. This is a hard cycle to break but you've already made a big step by realizing that you eat too much when you are sad.

What makes you happy? Visiting a friend? A long bubble bath? Exercising? Next time you feel sad, try a nonfood option for lifting your spirits. This is easier to suggest than to do, but now that you've identified a trigger for overeating you can change the behavior.

SMART STUFF—Exercise fights depression
Regular exercise releases natural brain chemicals (endorphins) that lift your spirits and make you feel happier.

Do I have to diet when I go out to eat with friends?

Dieters are very good at self-sabotage, finding excuses why they don't have to stick to their eating plan. You're smarter than that. In Chapter 6 and Chapter 11 we've given you loads of suggestions on how to eat out, eat well and have fun, too. It's not fun to go out with others and feel deprived. Instead of facing your night out with that attitude, look at the evening as an opportunity to practice thin habits and commonsense portions. The ultimate goal is to do this so effortlessly that none of your dinner companions will even know that you're dieting.

Instead of working on behavior changes, wouldn't it be simpler just to never eat chocolate cake again?

When a client asks a question like this, it's like watching a train wreck in slow motion; a disaster in the making. On the *Get Skinny* diet no foods are ever forbidden. We want you to take control of how much and how often you eat. Commonsense portions help you determine how much. How often depends on whether you've reached your target weight and how active you are. Active people burn more calories, so they can eat more.

While you're attempting to reach your target weight, chocolate cake definitely falls into the once-in-a-blue-moon category. Swearing an oath against eating future slices will most likely result in a chocolate cake binge somewhere in the not-too-distant future. If you don't binge, you'll be resentful, waiting for the day when you can eat chocolate cake again. You'll go off your diet, eat all the chocolate cake and other foods you gave up while dieting, and before you know it, you've gained back your lost weight.

Let's rewrite this scenario based on *Your Personalized Weight Attack Plan.* You love chocolate cake, so you decide you'll have a slice of chocolate cake every Saturday night. You also plan to take an extra long bike ride every weekend to help burn up the extra calories. We had a client who loved bagels with cream cheese. He enjoyed one, once a week, after his morning swim of one mile. On other days, he regularly swam 40 laps each morning, a little over half a mile. He traded the extra activity for a calorie dense choice. Don't deprive yourself, just plan.

Any ideas on how to avoid the office vending machines?

Short of never going near the vending machines, we'd suggest stocking your desk with snack choices that won't throw you off target. Fruit, individual bags of pretzels, calorie-reduced pudding, snack-pack fruit and fruit sauces, water, instant cereal, ready-to-eat sweetened cereal, single serving soups, even shelf stable yogurt can be kept without refrigeration. Add a small refrigerator and only your imagination will limit the choices.

The cafeteria lunch choices aren't helping my diet plan. Any suggestions?

Brown bag it. Bringing lunch from home is an easy way to cut down on impulsive choices on the cafeteria line. Though it may be time consuming at first, your efforts will be rewarded in calories saved and pounds lost.

How do I stop family and friends from urging me to eat when I shouldn't?

Dieting dynamics are interesting. When you're successfully controlling your weight the people around you often react in contradictory ways. Some become your cheerleader, celebrating each victory and reveling in your success. Others try to test your resolve by tempting you with foods you're trying to limit.

The husband of one of our clients brought her large boxes of candy to "celebrate" her weight loss. There was no stopping him. So she'd thank him profusely, eat one piece and take the rest of the box to work the next day. He finally got tired of buying her office mates candy and switched to buying his wife flowers.

Be firm with family members. Tell them how important it is for you to lose weight and how their support will make your job even easier. Friends who try to derail your eating plan may be jealous of your success. Interact with them less often for the time being. Good friends help, they don't hinder.

Because of our busy family schedule of drop-offs and pick-ups, some days if I don't eat in the car I won't get to eat. How do I handle this?

Eat at the table is a thin habit and we'd encourage you to do that as often as possible. But we also realize some days you'll have family obligations that must come first. Skipping a meal is never a good idea because you tend to overeat when you finally get a chance to eat. Plan for those car meals. Bring along good-for-you portable meals in a small cooler. Yogurt, fruit, salads, sandwiches, raw veggies, breadsticks, nonfat milk, cottage cheese, hard-cooked eggs, beans, and bottled water all travel well and many can be kept at room temperature. Make choices that will keep you on track when you're on-the-go.

There are nights when I just don't have the energy to cook a good meal. What then?

Assemble! The telephone and microwave are your two most indispensable kitchen tools. A take-out rotisserie chicken, bagged salad, microwave potatoes and ice pops for dessert requires no cooking and it's a good-for-the-whole-family meal. Order in—pizza with vegetables, no cheese; wonton soup with steamed shrimp and vegetables, plus a commonsense portion of brown rice. Don't fall into the trap of "if you don't cook dinner you won't eat well." Today, almost one-third of all meals eaten at home are warmed, not cooked.

What do I do if I can't find a minute to exercise?

Use everyday fitness to fill in the gap—clean the house, walk the dog, mow the lawn, rake leaves. Every 10-minute bout of activity counts. Watch TV and walk in place. It may sound silly but you are moving and burning calories. If walking in place is boring, do a strength training or stretching workout in front of the TV. Walk the halls at work after lunch. Jog on the overhead running track while your children play a game in the gym down below. Instead of taking the elevator, climb stairs between floors whenever possible. It can be a formal aerobics class or a bike ride to church; activity is simply building movement into your day.

How can I estimate the calories in a portion of food?

Not everything we eat comes with a nutrition label, that's why we set up *Get Skinny*'s commonsense portions and visual clues to help you "guesstimate" the calories in almost any food you are served. An average value for a cup of sliced fruit is 100 calories. You can use that figure for any fruit salad you eat. A yo-yo equals a mini bagel with approximately 100 calories. If your lunch sandwich comes on a roll, equal in size to 3 yo-yos, it has about 300 calories.

Another way to do it is to look up the calories in a similar food and use that value. For example, the calories in a slice of blueberry pie will be similar to the calories in a slice of apple pie. Though not 100% accurate, this shortcut will come close enough to keep you on target in your calorie zone.

I really don't like breakfast. Do I have to eat breakfast to lose weight?

Eat breakfast is a thin habit. Your body needs refueling in the morning. Without breakfast you burn calories less efficiently, actually making it harder to lose weight. Maybe what you hate are traditional breakfast foods. Be inventive. Have a smoothie. Swap breakfast and lunch choices. Try dinner leftovers. A sandwich? Pizza? An English muffin pizza made with a ¼ cup marinara sauce, 2 tablespoons of grated cheese and 2 tablespoons of sliced mushrooms has 225 calories. We're in favor of any choice that gets you to eat in the A.M.

I nibble when I cook. How can I stop?

You can nibble a few hundred extra calories while making dinner. Try chewing gum. It is unlikely that you will nibble with gum in your mouth.

You also need to look a little closer at why you are nibbling. Are you hungry? If so, try a midafternoon snack. A snack-size yogurt plus pectin would help blunt your pre-dinner hunger. Do you often skip lunch or don't eat enough at lunch? That sets you up for early evening hunger and may be the reason you're nibbling. Make yourself a salad or cut up a cup of raw vegetables and eat them while you're cooking as a pre-dinner appetizer. Nibbling doesn't have to sabotage your eating plan if you nibble the right choices.

What can I eat when I take the kids for hamburgers?

There isn't a child alive who doesn't enjoy, and expect, an occasional trip to the local hamburger spot with playgrounds, kid's meals and toys to collect. Though not the best place for a dieter, there are choices you can make and even enjoy without derailing your diet plan. Think commonsense portions and thin habits.

Order a regular hamburger, "undressed"; no cheese or special sauce. Top it with add-on's that won't add up—tomato slices, lettuce, mustard, salsa, pickle slices. Try grilled chicken sandwiches and a plain baked potato, when available. Instead of a milkshake, order lowfat chocolate milk. Skip the unlimited soda refills, unless you stick with diet soda. Order salad dressing on the side and use a commonsense portion. Even a "kid's meal" for Mom isn't a bad idea, because the portions are smaller.

SMART STUFF—Sampling counts

Sampling food from someone else's plate can add up. Each French fry = 11 calories.

Some days I just don't want to exercise. Is that okay?

Even elite athletes take days off. As long as you are reaching your weekly activity goal of using up a certain amount of calories, a day off every now and then is fine. The *Get Skinny* diet is about you and the lifestyle changes you're making to be slimmer and healthier. It's not boot camp. The only caution we'd add is don't take too many days off. This could derail your goals. Even when you feel tired, being active will invigorate you.

Getting Back on Track

You are painting yourself into the picture of a slimmer, fitter you. Occasionally you'll find yourself coloring outside the lines. When this happens:

- Take action immediately to get back to your target goals.
     One day of overeating or one day without activity does not make you a failure.
- Don't punish yourself for mistakes.
     Fasting, drastically cutting calories or adding an uncomfortable amount of exercise sets the stage for failure.

- Forget willpower, use strategies.

  The *Get Skinny* diet has armed you with powerful weapons—thin habits, commonsense portions, activity goals, hunger chasers, fat and calorie burners. Use them to win the diet war.

- Save one piece of clothing to remind you of your starting size.

  When you feel down, put it on to see how far you've already come.

- Appreciate that habits are hard to break but not impossible.

  Research has shown that changes in behavior are most effective when you are making those changes for yourself. Set your own goals; don't let someone else set them for you.

- Think about what, how and why you eat.

  To find the triggers that cause trouble you need to examine the links between emotions, situations and places that urge you to overeat.

- Watch the clock.

  Eating too often or going for long stretches without food are equally destructive, both causing you to eat too much. Many people need to build structure back into their eating plan with regular meals and snacks. Compare your usual eating pattern with the one we've suggested. Which is more satisfying?

- You count!

  Make your dieting goals and activity plan a priority. And don't always put yourself last.

Moving Along Menus

You'll use the **Moving Along** phase of *Get Skinny the Smart Way* until you reach your target weight. This phase will flow effortlessly into your lifetime eating plan. By the time you reach your target weight, you will be an expert in weight loss. Then in Chapter 11, You're in Charge, we'll give you even more tips and strategies to help you maintain your success.

Let's take a minute to assess where you are. Using **Smart Start**, you've lost a good amount of weight. You've integrated activity into your daily life and have increased your weekly activity goal. If you haven't already, you should be close to doubling your original activity goal. If you initially aimed to burn 750 calories a week, you should be edging close to 1500 calories burned each week through activity.

You now understand why we originally said that activity was a nonnegotiable part of *Your Personalized Weight Attack Plan*. It assures you quicker weight loss and it makes you feel good, not to mention look good. It probably feels a little odd now, to have a day when you aren't active. Yet, just a short time ago the reverse was true. It truly is time to "move along."

In the **Moving Along** phase of the *Get Skinny* diet you will be planning your day's menus. To get you started, we've given you a model for 1300, 1500, 1800 and 2000 calorie target zones. Use these or feel free to set up an individualized plan for your exact calorie zone and eating style.

Perhaps you no longer want 3 snacks a day. Fine, just don't go for long stretches without eating. Maybe you'd rather have your largest meal at lunch to accommodate business obligations. That's a good switch. Maybe you've started to add pectin to other foods so you are going to drop the A.M. yogurt–pectin hunger chaser. That's okay, just remember pectin is a strong weight loss ally, so keep using it.

An eating plan for 1300 to 1500 calories a day will rely more on the less calorie dense choices in each of the commonsense food categories. For example, choosing leaner meat, fish and poultry, which are less calorie dense than those with more fat, skin or breading. Eating plans for 1800 and 2000 calories a day allow greater use of some of the more calorie dense options. That doesn't mean that you can never eat prime rib if you are on a 1300 calorie plan. It simply means you need to "plan" to eat prime rib. When a more calorie dense choice is made it needs to be balanced with other less calorie dense choices to keep you on track in your target calorie zone.

Our primary goal with the *Get Skinny* diet was to put you in charge of your eating plan. We're ready for you to take over, so let's get started.

The Basics

The **Moving Along** menu plan incorporates healthy eating principles. Each day's menu includes:

- 2 calcium-rich foods a day
- 5 commonsense servings of fruits and vegetables
- 4 or more commonsense servings of breads, cereals and other grains
- at least 4 ounces of meat, fish, poultry or other protein foods

Depending on your personalized calorie zone and your individualized weekly activity goal, you may to able to add more servings, snacks, add-ons or sweets to your **Moving Along** menus.

In addition to planning your daily menu, each day you need to:

- take a 600 milligram calcium supplement
- drink 8 to 10 glasses of water or other fluids
- add 1 to 3 teaspoons of pectin to foods to make you feel fuller longer
- select fiber-rich foods whenever possible
- track your activity on your Weekly Activity Log

We'd also recommend that you use your Daily Food Diary 2 to 3 times during each week of **Moving Along** to be sure you stay on target.

Moving Along Menu Plans

The **Moving Along** menu plans are set up for 1300, 1500, 1800 and 2000 target calorie zones. We've provided a model for each target calorie zone and a worksheet for you to write in the specific foods you've chosen. You can either use these menu models or set up your own individualized plan for your calorie zone and eating style. As long as you track your calories 2 to 3 times a week, using your Daily Food Diary, either system will work.

GET SKINNY AT A GLANCE

It's hard to remember everything about eating well and being active, so here is a quick reference when you need a refresher. To learn more about:

The menu models have been planned using the calorie values from commonsense portions. These are average figures. If you track your calories more precisely, using the values found in Appendix 3, you may be able to eat more of some foods or use the extra calories for add-ons or treats.

Target Calorie Zone
1300 Calories

Breakfast	Commonsense Portion
Bread, ready-to-eat cereal, waffle	1
Nonfat milk	1 cup
Fresh fruit	1 cup
All fruit jelly	1 tablespoon
Calorie-free beverage	

A.M. Snack
Yogurt + pectin	1 snack size

Lunch
Bread	1
Lean protein	2 ounces
Tossed salad	2 cups
Reduced-calorie salad dressing	2 tablespoons
Calorie-free beverage	

Afternoon Snack
Fresh fruit	1 medium

Dinner
Lean meat, fish or poultry	4 ounces
Potato, corn, peas, sweet potato, winter squash, plantain	1 cup or 1 medium
Steamed vegetables	1 cup
Calorie-free beverage	

P.M. Snack
Snack of choice for 50 calories or less

Target Calorie Zone
1300 Calories

Breakfast   **Commonsense Portion**
_____   _____
_____   _____
_____   _____
_____   _____
_____

A.M. Snack
_____   _____

Lunch
_____   _____
_____   _____
_____   _____
_____   _____

Afternoon Snack
_____   _____

Dinner
_____   _____
_____   _____
_____   _____
_____

P.M. Snack
_____   _____

Target Calorie Zone
1500 Calories

Breakfast	Commonsense Portion
Bread, ready-to-eat cereal, waffle	1
Nonfat milk	1 cup
Fresh fruit	1 cup
All fruit jelly	1 tablespoon
Calorie-free beverage	

A.M. Snack

Yogurt + pectin	1 snack size

Lunch

Bread	2
Lean protein	2 ounces
Tossed salad	2 cups
Reduced-calorie salad dressing	2 tablespoons
Calorie-free beverage	

Afternoon Snack

Fresh fruit	1 medium

Dinner

Lean meat, fish or poultry	4 ounces
Rice, beans or baked potato	1 cup or 1 medium
Steamed vegetables	1 cup
Calorie-free beverage	

P.M. Snack

Snack of choice for 75 calories or less

Target Calorie Zone
1500 Calories

Breakfast

_____
_____
_____
_____
_____

A.M. Snack

_____

Lunch

_____
_____
_____
_____
_____

Afternoon Snack

_____

Dinner

_____
_____
_____
_____

P.M. Snack

_____

Commonsense Portion

_____
_____
_____
_____
_____

_____

_____
_____
_____
_____

_____

_____
_____
_____
_____

_____

Target Calorie Zone
1800 Calories

Breakfast	Commonsense Portion
Bread, ready-to-eat cereal, waffle	2
Nonfat milk	1 cup
Fresh fruit	1 cup
All fruit jelly	1 tablespoon
Calorie-free beverage	

A.M. Snack

Yogurt + pectin	1 regular size

Lunch

Bread	2
Lean protein	2 ounces
Tossed salad	2 cups
Reduced-calorie salad dressing	2 tablespoons
Calorie-free beverage	

Afternoon Snack

Fresh fruit	1 medium

Dinner

Moderately lean meat, fish or poultry	4 ounces
Rice, beans or baked potato	1 cup or 1 medium
Steamed vegetables	1 cup
Calorie-free beverage	

P.M. Snack

Snack of choice for less than 125 calories

Target Calorie Zone
1800 Calories

Breakfast   **Commonsense Portion**
_____   _____
_____   _____
_____   _____
_____   _____
_____

A.M. **Snack**
_____   _____

Lunch
_____   _____
_____   _____
_____   _____
_____   _____
_____

Afternoon Snack
_____   _____

Dinner
_____   _____
_____   _____
_____   _____
_____   _____
_____

P.M. **Snack**
_____   _____

Target Calorie Zone
2000 Calories

Breakfast	**Commonsense Portion**
Bread, ready-to-eat cereal, waffle	2
Nonfat milk	1 cup
Fresh fruit	1 cup
All fruit jelly	1 tablespoon
Whipped margarine	1 tablespoon
Calorie-free beverage	

A.M. Snack	
Yogurt + pectin	1 regular size

Lunch	
Bread	2
Lean protein	2 ounces
Tossed salad	2 cups
Reduced-calorie salad dressing	2 tablespoons
Calorie-free beverage	

Afternoon Snack	
Fresh fruit	1 medium

Dinner	
Moderately lean meat, fish or poultry	4 ounces
Rice, beans or baked potato	1 cup or 1 medium
Steamed vegetables	1 cup
Bread or small dinner roll	1
Whipped margarine	1 tablespoon
Calorie-free beverage	

P.M. Snack

Snack of choice for less than 125 calories

Target Calorie Zone
2000 Calories

Breakfast   **Commonsense Portion**
_____   _____
_____   _____
_____   _____
_____   _____
_____   _____

A.M. Snack
_____   _____

Lunch
_____   _____
_____   _____
_____   _____
_____

Afternoon Snack
_____   _____

Dinner
_____   _____
_____   _____
_____   _____
_____   _____

P.M. Snack
_____   _____

Moving Along Recipes

On the next few pages are a few more quick, tasty, low calorie recipes to help tweak your imagination while you're planning your **Moving Along** menus. Each recipe gives the calories in one serving to help you stay in your target calorie zone.

Couscous Tuna Salad

1 cup water
⅔ cup couscous
1 large red pepper, seeded and chopped (about 1½ cups)
2 cucumbers, peeled and chopped (about 1½ cups)
1 medium onion, chopped (about 1 cup)
½ cup raisins
1 can (11 ounces) corn, drained
1 can (6 ounces) tuna in water, drained and flaked
¼ cup reduced-calorie italian dressing

Bring 1 cup water to boil, add couscous, stir and let stand 5 minutes. In a large bowl toss all ingredients to combine. Makes 10 servings.

1 serving = 1 cup   173 calories

Curried Chicken & Vegetables

2½ cups nonfat milk
1 can (10 ounces) reduced fat cream soup
1 bag (1 pound) frozen mixed vegetables
2 cups (any shape) pasta
1 package (10 ounces) ready-to-eat chicken
½ to 1 teaspoon curry powder

In a large saucepan stir milk and soup to combine. Bring to a boil, stir in pasta and cook 5 minutes; add vegetables and cook 5 additional minutes or until pasta and vegetables are tender. Add chicken and curry powder, let stand 5 minutes for flavors to blend and chicken to warm. Makes 4 servings.

1 serving   273 calories

Chicken in Mushroom Gravy

4 boneless chicken breasts (about 1 pound)
1 can (10 ounces) lowfat cream soup
½ can water
1 can (4 ounces) sliced mushrooms, drained

Coat a frying pan with nonstick cooking spray. Brown chicken breasts on both sides for about 2 minutes. Combine soup and water, stirring until smooth. Add soup and mushrooms to pan, bring to a boil, reduce heat to low, cover and cook 10 minutes. Makes 4 servings.

1 serving = 1 chicken breast + gravy   125 calories

Oven Roasted Fries

Garlic flavored nonstick cooking spray
4 potatoes, scrubbed and cut into strips
Paprika

Preheat oven to 425°F. Spray a shallow baking pan with nonstick cooking spray. Place potatoes on pan in a single layer. Lightly spray potatoes with cooking spray and sprinkle with paprika. Bake for 20 minutes or until potatoes are fork tender. Makes 4 servings.

1 serving = 1 cup (about 10 pieces)   150 calories

Quick Pasta e Fagiole

3 cloves garlic, minced
1 teaspoon dried rosemary
2 cans (14 ounces each) chicken broth
1 cup water
2 cans (14 ounces each) diced tomatoes, Italian style
1 cup ditallini pasta (or other small-shaped pasta), uncooked
1 can (15 ounces) white or cannelloni beans, drained and rinsed

Coat a large pot with nonstick cooking spray. Add garlic and rosemary and cook, stirring constantly for 1 minute. Add broth, water, tomatoes and pasta. Bring to a boil, reduce heat to medium (a gentle boil) and cook for 10 minutes. Add beans and continue cooking 2 to 3 minutes longer until beans are heated. To serve, sprinkle each bowl of soup with ½ teaspoon grated parmesan cheese and fresh pepper. Makes 5 servings.

1 serving = 2 cups   260 calories

Savory Bolognese Pasta Sauce

½ pound extra lean ground beef
2 cans (14 ounces each) Italian-flavored diced tomatoes
1 cup grated carrot
2 tablespoons balsamic vinegar

Coat a large frying pan with nonstick cooking spray. Brown ground beef over high heat until it has lost its pink color. Add tomatoes, carrot and vinegar; cover, reduce heat to low and cook 10 minutes. Makes 5 cups.

1 serving = 1 cup sauce (151 calories) + 2 cups cooked pasta (400 calories)

1 serving   551 calories

One-Dish Seafood Dinner

2½ cups water
1 cup kasha (buckwheat groats)
1 package (6 ounces) frozen pea pods
¼ cup sliced scallions
1 package (16 ounces) frozen crab substitute
1 tablespoon light soy sauce

In a large saucepan bring water and kasha to a boil; reduce heat to low, cover and cook 10 minutes. Add scallions, pea pods and shellfish substitute; continue cooking 2 to 3 minutes until heated through. Makes 6 servings.

1 serving   164 calories

Slow-Cooked Barbecue Beef

1 large onion, chopped
1 tablespoon cider vinegar
1 can (4.5 ounces) green chilies, chopped
1 package (1.25 ounces) taco seasoning mix
1 (1½ pound) London broil

Coat an electric slow cooker with nonstick cooking spray. Add onion, vinegar and chilies. Trim any fat from meat. Sprinkle half the taco mix into the slow cooker, add meat and sprinkle remaining taco mix on top of meat. Cover and let cook 7 to 8 hours. Shred cooked meat by pulling apart with two forks (it will be exceedingly tender). Serve over cooked rice or on a whole wheat hamburger bun.

Makes 6 servings   1 serving = 242 calories

Fisherman's Stew

1 stalk celery, chopped
24 baby carrots
1 can (14 ounces) chicken broth
1 cup frozen pearl onions
8 new red potatoes, scrubbed and halved
1 pound cod steak

Spray a large frying pan with nonstick cooking spray. Fry celery and baby carrots 2 to 3 minutes until celery begins to soften. Add broth, onions, potatoes and cod. Bring to a boil, cover, reduce heat to simmer and cook 10 minutes until fish flakes and potatoes are tender. Makes 4 servings.

1 serving   237 calories

Chapter 11

You're in Control—
Maintaining Your Success

> . . . it is the responsibility of obesity researchers to tell the public that they really need to think about food and exercise all the time.
>
> —Dr. James Hill, Obesity Researcher,
> University of Colorado

The day you have been working toward has finally arrived. You've reached your target weight! As excited as you are, the big question looming in your head is, "Now what?". The answer is, "You're in charge." You made the weight loss happen. You became fitter by being more active. You are in control and you can stay that way.

The biggest problem with most diets is that they end. At that point, without the structure of the diet to follow, a person often goes back to old eating habits that got them into trouble in the first place. The *Get Skinny* diet doesn't end. It eases you into control. And that's where you are right now. You own all the tools needed to be slimmer and more active. They have become part of your daily routine. Just continue to:

- Use thin habits.
- Eat commonsense portions.

- Get adequate calcium.
- Drink enough water and other fluids each day.
- Rely on your pectin hunger chaser if you need it.
- Keep moving.

Steer Clear of the Hard Sell

If you paid attention to the majority of television commercials you see in a day, you'd head straight for the couch with a bag of potato chips or a piping hot pizza, washed down with a can of soda. Fats, oils, sweets and beverages rank as the most highly advertised foods, with fruits and vegetables trailing far behind, averaging only 5% of advertisement spots.

Luckily, we're a savvy bunch who treat most advertisements with a healthy dose of skepticism. But lurking not far behind is a more subtle and insidious influence. Your favorite TV characters are rarely shown exercising, yet they eat and drink to abandon. Few, if any, are overweight or face major chronic health problems like heart disease, diabetes or cancer. And we're told the media mimics real life. Where weight control and exercise are concerned, we don't think so!

Just knowing these subliminal messages are out there, waiting to trip you up, is enough to stop them from influencing your behavior.

SMART STUFF
A research study showed that TV comedy shows, which attract the biggest family audiences, had the largest number of references to less healthy foods.

Trade "Cheat" for "Negotiate"

Dieter's love to cheat. On *Your Personalized Weight Attack Plan,* you'll never need to cheat again because *no foods are forbidden.* Now that you are at your target weight, there are probably some favorites you'd like to eat more often than you did when you were actively trying to lose. That's fine. A commonsense portion of any food is a good food.

Keeping portion sizes reasonable and relegating some very calorie dense choices, like hot fudge sundaes and fried chicken, to the once-in-a-blue-moon category will keep you from eating too much too often. Let's look at ways to negotiate choices that may have tempted you to cheat in the past.

Love Chocolate?

You're not alone. Forty percent of women and 15% of men say they sometimes crave chocolate. Actually, chocolate is good for you. It contains many of the same antioxidants found in red wine that lower your risk for heart disease. Men who regularly eat chocolate and other candy live almost a year longer than those who don't and this benefit is consistent up to age 95.

The biggest problem with chocolate is that it can be a calorie dense food, but not always. Instead of a solid chocolate bar, try a chocolate-covered wafer cookie, graham cracker, pretzels or mints with soft centers. A fudgesicle or chocolate Italian ice can replace rich chocolate ice cream. Reduced-calorie chocolate syrup, made with cocoa powder and sugar, warmed in the microwave, can substitute for more calorie dense hot fudge. Chocolate meringue cookies and chocolate rice cakes are low calorie snacks. A chocolate Tootsie Pop delivers long-lasting taste for less than half the calories of a solid chocolate bar. And, for those times when nothing but the real thing will do, have a snack size of your favorite.

SMART START—When you get the urge for an ice cream sundae

Start with lowfat frozen yogurt or reduced-calorie ice cream. Spoon on pureed raspberries or crushed pineapple. Top with marshmallow fluff or reduced-calorie whipped topping. Sprinkle with "sprinkles." And don't forget the cherry!

Have Favorites Au Naturel

Eat slowly, and *chew, it's satisfying,* are two thin habits. Anything that slows down eating is a positive behavior.

Enjoy shrimp "in the shell." Peeling them slows you down and you'll eat less of them. Dipping the shrimp into cocktail sauce adds a few extra calories, but a squeeze of lemon is calorie free.

Eat whole, steamed artichokes, leaf by leaf. They're delicious, time-consuming and fun. Spray with calorie-free butter spray instead of dipping the leaves into melted butter.

Eat a whole orange or grapefruit by peeling off the skin and separating the sections, one by one. It will take you far longer to eat than downing a quick glass of juice and you'll get added fiber, as well.

When was the last time you ate green peas from the shell? In season, fresh raw peas make a sweet, crunchy, low calorie snack. A year-round alternative is edamame, fresh soybeans in a shell. You'll find them in the freezer at your local supermarket. They cook quickly and have an interesting nutty taste.

Even peanuts in the shell can fit into your sensible eating plan. Twenty-four peanuts will take a long time to crack and eat but they yield a scant 2 tablespoons of nuts. The same applies to seeds. A quarter cup of sunflower kernels has the same calories as three quarters of a cup of sunflower seeds. A small bonus—you'll burn a few calories shelling while you eat.

Good Things Come in Small Packages

Buy single-servings, and *small sizes = smaller you,* are two thin habits that encourage you to trade taste for size.

Choose	Instead of	Calories Saved
Snack-size chocolate bar	Regular chocolate bar	184
Bite-size chocolate covered mint	Chocolate covered mint patty	210
Snack-size bag potato chips	Regular 6-ounce bag chips	750
Chocolate cupcake with icing	Slice of chocolate layer cake	282

(continued)

Good Things Come in Small Packages (cont.)

Choose	Instead of	Calories Saved
Cheesecake snack bar	Slice of cheesecake	306
Crispy rice bar	Large take-out cookie	200
1 scoop ice cream in wafer cone	4-scoop waffle cone	637
Small hamburger	Double patty burger with cheese	269
4-ounce filet mignon	10-ounce Porterhouse steak	612
10-ounce can soda	Value-size (32 ounce) soda	277
10-ounce small coffee with sugar and cream	16-ounce large coffee with sugar and cream	60
3-ounce frozen bagel	5-ounce take-out bagel	200
2 large hard pretzels	1 large soft pretzel	225
1 cup chicken noodle soup	1 bowl chicken noodle soup	90

Sweet Endings

There are times when you could die for something sweet to eat. We hate diets that tell you to have "just one bite," because we know from experience that, for most people, that will rarely do. *Eat slowly,* and *chew, it's satisfying,* are two thin habits that work, even with sweets. A commonsense portion of a sweet indulgence—a quarter of a cup—gives you enough to savor without feeling cheated. We recommend sweets that come in small pieces, which you can eat one or two at a time.

A Piece, Not a Handful

Sweet & Treats	Calories in ¼ Cup
Candy corn	216
Chocolate covered peanuts	193
Chocolate covered raisins	185
Chocolate coated mini mints	180
Gumdrops	135

Sweet & Treats	Calories in ¼ Cup
Jelly beans	150
Lemon drops, hard candy (8)	160
Malted milk balls (8)	130
Mini milk chocolate bars (4)	184
Mini marshmallows	50
Mini peanut butter cups (4)	168
Party mints	90

Knowing you can negotiate a commonsense portion of any food into *Your Personalized Weight Attack Plan,* you'll never have to consider "cheating" again.

A Little Insanity Is Normal

A day when your eating goes out of control will cause you some immediate regret. But lasting weight gain? Unlikely. Everybody has a day, every now and then, when they eat too much. Most people believe they've gained pounds from this misadventure. But the truth is, they haven't. They may be up a few ounces but, with sensible eating plus activity, this will come off in the next few days.

Not convinced? You know that the day after eating too much, when you get on your scale, you often see a weight gain of 2 to 3 pounds. We're talking ounces; you see pounds.

Theoretically, if you eat 3500 extra calories, you should gain a pound. Even on your best overeating day, 3500 extra calories is a lot. Especially since you're now a much more sensible eater. Your current binges aren't nearly as devastating as you think. Secondly, the calories you eat don't automatically go to your hips and belly. Many are burned off as heat and many are used to keep your body functioning. Some will be stored as fat, to be used in the future. If this storage goes unused, over time it will mount up to added weight. You're clear on this explanation but you still don't understand where the morning-after weight gain came from.

Often the foods you overindulge in are high in carbohydrates (pasta), sugars (dessert) and sodium (most food eaten away from home). All of these tend to make you retain water. So the morning-after weight gain is mostly fluid retention, which will disappear over the next couple of days.

Dr. Kelly Brownell, professor of psychology at Yale University, believes the biggest message here is not to "turn a little detour into a catastrophe." If you have an out-of-control eating day, say "oops" and get right back on track eating commonsense portions and being active. You can't do much damage from one detour.

Enlarging Your Repertoire

Dried fruits, nuts and fruit juices have not been a part of the *Get Skinny* diet while you were working toward your target weight. All are good-for-you choices that are somewhat calorie dense.

Fruit juices offer no chewing, so you can swallow many more calories in a mouthful. Try diluting your favorite with seltzer or mineral water to add more fluid and cut the calories. Fruit juice and fruit nectar ice cubes can add flavor and nutrients to water, seltzer or even diet soda, lemonade and iced tea. Keep some handy in the freezer.

Dried fruits have the same calories as the fresh fruit from which they came. In the dried variety, with water removed, the calories and natural sugars are packed into a smaller but sweeter serving size. Twenty raisins have the same calories as 20 grapes. The raisins barely fill up a tablespoon but the grapes equal nearly 1 cup. Dried fruits are portable, nutritious and sweet. A quarter cup is a commonsense portion, but grabbing handful after handful is not the way to go.

Nuts are rich in monounsaturated oil, similar to heart-healthy olive oil. Research has shown that eating moderate amounts could reduce your risk for heart disease. But, like dried fruits, many calories come packed in a small serving. So measure, don't grab.

Measure, Don't Grab

Dried Fruit	Count in ¼ cup	Calories in ¼ cup
Apricot halves	8	96
Cranberries	60	98
Dates	5–6	110
Figs	5–6	100
Plums (prunes)	6	100
Raisins	80–90	109
Nuts		
Almonds		170
Cashews		170
Mixed nuts		180
Peanuts		170
Pine nuts		140
Pistachios		160
Trail mix		170
Walnuts, halves		170
Wasabi peanuts		150

Top 10—So There's Always Something to Eat

You come home after a long day and the last thing on your mind is what's for dinner. But you're hungry. You start rummaging around the kitchen and, before your know it, you've nibbled on this and taken a few bites of that.

By keeping a few basics on hand you'll never again groan "there's nothing to eat!" Here's our "top 10" cabinet stuffers. Feel free to add your favorites.

1. Flavor boosters

Taste is the number one reason we choose foods. All of these pack flavor—some with no calories, others with a few. Keep a selection on hand to add a flavor punch to quick meals. Look in Chapter 8 for more ideas on how to use them.

Just Taste, No Calories	Lots of Taste, a Few Calories
Balsamic vinegar	Ketchup
Flavored vinegar	All fruit jelly
Cooking and butter spray	Reduced-calorie salad dressing
Cracked pepper	Anchovy paste
Hot sauce	Spiked sherry
Horseradish	
Lemons	
Light soy sauce	
Mustard	
Salsa	
Worcestershire sauce	

2. **Seasoned, canned, diced tomatoes**

This is our favorite canned food and you'll find it in many of the recipes throughout this book. Depending on the brand, you'll find Italian, chili, garlic, basil or onion flavored varieties, most available in 14-ounce cans.

Mix with leftovers and instant rice for a quick Spanish rice. Add cooked chicken and shrimp and you have a main dish. You can be equally inventive with pasta. As little as a quarter pound of cooked, crumbled chopped beef or ground turkey, plus flavored tomatoes over pasta, makes dinner in the time it takes to cook the pasta. Add a dash of sherry pepper and you'll be impressed with your creation. Use seasoned tomatoes as the liquid to "poach" any fish fillets. Pour the tomatoes into a shallow pan with a lid, place the fish on top, bring to a simmer, cover and cook for 10 minutes or until fish flakes. Choose a flavor booster to put your imprint on this dish.

3. **Broth—chicken, beef or vegetable**

Available canned, in shelf-stable cardboard boxes, or dried. Alone, broth offers a soothing, low calorie warm drink when you need to shift gears or just relax. Some brands are available fat free (even though the fat calories are minimal in all varieties), lower in sodium, or flavored with roasted garlic or onions for even more taste.

Use broth to replace part of the water when making rice, couscous, kasha, instant mashed potatoes, or stuffing mixes. Because broth packs flavor, you can leave out the butter or oil called for on the package directions, adding flavor while cutting calories. And broth can be the base for clean-out-the-refrigerator night. A little leftover pasta, some vegetables and cooked chicken, makes a soup in no time. When no chicken or meat is in the fridge, open a can of beans for a hearty main dish soup. Or invent your own soup with noodles and frozen vegetables.

4. **Yogurt**

Available nonfat or reduced fat plain and flavored or snack-size, it must be pretty obvious by now that we are yogurt fans. Besides providing you with an instant base for your pectin hunger chaser, it's an important source of calcium.

A container of yogurt can be turned into a meal when topped with wheat germ, granola or a spoonful of nuts and accompanied by a fruit salad. It's also a great stretcher—add some plain nonfat yogurt to regular mayonnaise, tartar sauce, sour cream or salad dressings for the same taste you enjoy with less calories. Plain yogurt can also be used to top foods traditionally dressed with sour cream—tacos, fajitas, baked potatoes—or used in recipes that call for sour cream as an ingredient.

5. **Bagged salad**

We don't think it's silly that you are so time-stressed you can't cut up a salad. Keeping mixed salads or cut-up, ready-to-use salad ingredients in the fridge is a true time saver. You're more likely to have salad often if it's easy to make. Adding a hard-cooked egg, canned tuna, canned salmon, ready-to-eat chicken, deli ham or roast beef, turns a side salad into a meal. It's also a filling, low calorie addition to a wrap sandwich.

6. **Frozen vegetables**

Like salad, if time is an issue, shopping for and cutting up fresh vegetables doesn't always fit into your day. Let bags of frozen vegetables come to your rescue. Whether individual or in combos, the variety available is endless and constantly changing. All cook quickly in the microwave and this method of preparation has frozen rivaling fresh for taste and crispness. Gone are the days of water-logged, soggy, pale vegetables.

Only your imagination will limit the use of this kitchen basic. Eat favorites along with dinner. Throw a cup or two into pasta during the last few minutes of cooking as the basis for a pasta primavera meal. Add them when cooking rice to invent a pilaf. Use them as the base for a stir-fry dish. Or drizzle your favorite with reduced-calorie salad dressing for a vegetable salad. Low in calories, rich in nutrients and fiber, there are few things you could choose that are better for you.

7. **Canned tuna or chicken**

Canned tuna is a staple in most kitchens but canned chicken may be something new to you. Available in broth and found near the tuna on the supermarket shelf, it offers equal versatility as a lean protein. Both come in different can sizes. Tuna can be found in flip-top individual to family-size cans. Packed in water is best but if you prefer oil-packed, simply drain off the oil and you'll be eating a commonsense portion of a moderately lean protein choice.

Both can be added to pasta, rice, salad, stir fried with vegetables, eaten in a pita or wrap, or added to a lowfat cream soup for "à la king." Try either with some chopped scallions, celery and cucumber plus a drizzle of reduced-calorie salad dressing on a bed of your favorite bagged salad mix.

8. **Frozen turkey or garden (vegetable/soy) burgers**

These are quick-cooking, leaner, portion controlled alternatives to the traditional hamburger. Dressed like a hamburger, you'll be hard-pressed to tell them from the real thing. Check out the supermarket freezer case—new brands and new flavors are constantly popping up, a tribute to how good these products can be.

The classic way to serve these burgers is on a roll or as a meat substitute, but they can be crumbled into pasta sauce or creamed soup, or added to rice, couscous or pasta mixes as part of a one-dish meal.

9. **Grains—pasta, rice, couscous, kasha**

Pick your favorites and keep a few on hand. Grains are the base for any meal. Served hot as a main dish they are savory; served cold as the base for a salad, they're zesty. Every other "favorite" we've listed so far goes with grains. Try stirring nonfat plain yogurt into warm marinara sauce to make a "pink sauce." Add a dash of vodka for "pasta à la vodka."

10. **Beans, regular or fat free refried**

Canned beans are easy to find but the freezer case in the supermarket also has a growing frozen variety. Like meat, beans, which are low in fat and high in fiber, can be added to salad, soups, combo dishes, pita or wraps.

Fat free refried beans are one of our favorites. Straight from the can they can be heated as a side dish. Add a little diced Canadian bacon for a smokier flavor. Spread some on a wrap with crunchy toppers, nonfat yogurt and flavor boosters of your choice for an interesting lunch alternative. Or mix with salsa to make a dip for crackers and fresh vegetables.

Keep Moving

Remaining active after you reach your target weight is like opening a savings account. Instead of banking money, you're saving calories. At this point the calories you burn up through activity will compensate for foods you wish to eat more often than you did when you were trying to lose. Now it's okay to add a dinner roll at supper. You're still active and at your target weight. So the activity burns up the calories from the dinner roll. Without activity, the 100 calories from the roll might be just that little extra that starts adding up.

Activity speeds up your metabolism and builds muscle, and both help you burn calories quicker. Studies done on people who maintained their successful weight loss for years were active several times a week. When life gets busy and you skip activity for a day or even a week or two, don't feel defeated. The benefits of exercise don't disappear overnight; it would actually take months to lose all you've achieved. A little time off is just an "oops." Simply pick up where you left off and get moving again.

Exercise makes you slimmer, healthier and lifts your spirits. Why wouldn't you want to be thinner, healthier and happier?

SMART STUFF—The power of change

As you practice new eating habits, your tastes will change. Food that once seemed delicious may begin to taste too sweet, too salty or too fatty. Some good-for-you substitutes may become your new idea of heaven on earth

Chapter 12

Take a Bow—
You're Picture Perfect!

> It takes knowledge, motivation, action and time to
> create change.

You are the picture of success! You've reached your targets. Your plate is picture perfect! Your weight is on target or close to it! Your health is improved! You're moving and enjoying it! Look into the mirror—you'll like that person smiling back.

No one would argue that a fit, energetic, slimmer person is the "picture of health." As you changed your eating and activity behavior you, quite literally, changed your life. You painted a new picture of you. Let's take a minute to see what that picture looks like, shall we?

Painting Your Picture of Health

Circle the answer that best applies to you.

Your Plate Is Picture Perfect

1. I eat meals and snacks at regular intervals throughout the day.
   A. Every day
   B. Almost every day
   C. Most days

2. I eat breakfast.
   A. Every day
   B. Almost every day
   C. Most days (less than 5 days a week)

3. I drink enough fluids each day.
   A. 8 to 10 cups
   B. At least 8 cups
   C. Less than 8 cups. I'm still working on this behavior.

4. I eat whole grain breads, cereals, rice or pasta.
   A. Almost always
   B. Most of the time
   C. Often. I'm still working on this behavior.

5. I eat 5 servings of fruits and vegetables each day.
   A. Every day
   B. Almost every day
   C. Often. I'm still working on this behavior.

6. I eat at least 2 excellent sources of calcium each day (milk, yogurt, calcium-fortified soy milk, calcium-fortified juice, reduced fat cheese).
   A. Every day
   B. Almost every day
   C. Often. I'm still working on this behavior.

7. I choose reduced-calorie or whipped varieties of margarine, mayonnaise, cream cheese, sour cream, cream and salad dressing.
   A. Always
   B. Almost always
   C. Occasionally

8. I almost always choose:
   A. Nonfat milk
   B. 1% milk
   C. 2% milk

9. I choose reduced fat or nonfat frozen yogurt and ice cream:
   A. Always
   B. Almost always
   C. Occasionally

10. I limit beer, wine, and liquor to no more than 1 drink a day for women and 2 drinks a day for men.
    A. Always
    B. Almost always
    C. Often. I'm still working on this behavior.

11. I use thin habits to help me eat well.
    A. Always
    B. Almost always
    C. Most of the time. I'm still working on this behavior.

12. I eat commonsense portions.
    A. Always
    B. Almost always
    C. Most of the time. I'm still working on this behavior.

13. I eat when I'm hungry and stop when I feel full.
    A. Always
    B. Almost always
    C. Often. I'm still working on this behavior.

14. I eat late in the evening or in the middle of the night.
    A. Never
    B. Almost never
    C. Once in a while. I'm still working on this behavior.

15. I find non-food options to channel my emotions.
    A. Almost all the time
    B. Usually
    C. Sometimes. I'm still working on this behavior.

You Look Picture Perfect

16. My current weight is:
    A. At my target weight
    B. Going down and less than 5 pounds from my target weight
    C. Going down

17. My BMI (Body Mass Index) is:
    A. Below 25
    B. At 25
    C. Above 25 but coming down

18. My current activity level is:
    A. Double my original weekly activity goal
    B. Close to double my original weekly activity goal
    C. Good. I'm still working toward being more active.

19. I participate in at least 30 minutes of activity (walking, running, swimming, dancing, exercise classes, bicycling, rollerblading, basketball).
    A. Every day
    B. 4 to 6 times a week
    C. 2 to 3 times a week

20. I participate in stretching exercises, yoga or tai chi.
    A. 3 or more times a week
    B. At least 2 times a week
    C. Sometimes. I'm still working on this behavior.

21. I participate in strength training exercises (free weights or resistance machines)
    A. 3 or more times a week
    B. At least 2 times a week
    C. Sometimes. I'm still working on this behavior.

22. I enjoy recreational sports activities (golf, tennis, volleyball, dancing, table tennis).
    A. At least twice a week
    B. At least once a week
    C. Sometimes. I'm still working on this behavior.

23. I use exercise to reduce stress and relax.
    A. Almost always
    B. As often as I can
    C. Sometimes. I'm still working on this behavior.

24. I practice good health habits, like flossing my teeth, using sun screen and wearing seat belts.

A. Every day
B. Almost every day
C. Most of the time. I'm still working on this behavior.

Your Picture of Health

This is a test you can't fail because every answer indicates a change for the better in how you eat and in your activity level.

A—**A**chieving your goal
B—**B**etter than you'd ever hoped for
C—**C**oming Close to Changing a behavior

Add up the number of As, Bs and Cs you circled and write them below.

A answers _____   B answers _____   C answers _____

"A" answers show you've made positive changes in your eating or activity behaviors. "B" answers show you've changed your eating and activity behaviors for the better. There is still a little room for improvement but you've come a long, long way from where you started. Even with "C" answers you are still a winner. As we've said, from the beginning it's hard to change many things at once. But you are changing and that's what counts.

Every so often go back and see how your portrait is coming along. Again, don't expect to change overnight. But remember, every positive change you make will have a positive impact on maintaining your weight, improving your health and reducing your stress.

SMART STUFF—Good food, bad food?
Media messages often label foods "bad" or "good." A commonsense portion of any food, once in a while—hamburgers, cake, ice cream, fudge—is not "bad." Likewise, an apple or two, sandwiched among otherwise questionable choices, is not "good."

Your Game Plan

According to behavioral science researchers, successful change has several stages from:

- "I have no thoughts about changing my life"—precontemplation stage

   The old inactive, heavier you.

      to

- "I'll think about changing"—contemplation stage

   You began to think seriously about changing your eating behavior when you bought *Get Skinny the Smart Way* and brought it home. In this stage you made a tremendous psychological jump from "No, way, not me!" to "I'll give it some thought."

      to

- "I'm ready for change"—preparation stage

   You were finally ready for action at this point. You started to read *Get Skinny the Smart Way* and began to assess your eating and activity.

      to

- "I'm changing"—action stage

   You worked your way through **Smart Start** and **Moving Along**, you met your activity goals and you reached your target weight.

      and, finally,

- "I want to keep the ball rolling"—maintenance stage

   You see yourself slimmer, healthier and more active and you want to stay that way.

Even though you may not have consciously recognized these behavioral stages, you set up your own game plan for healthy living and moved through it. In some behavior chains there is a termination stage, where change has occurred and no further action is required. That's the spot where many successful dieters get into trouble.

Dieting doesn't have a termination stage. Instead, you'll stay in maintenance—"keeping the ball rolling"—indefinitely. And you'll be successful. Facing food and making the right choices, and being active almost every day, are part of who you are now. You own these behaviors and have integrated them into your life. Just keep on doing what you're doing.

SMART STUFF
Self-esteem is calorie free.

Check and Balance

Successful long-term weight management is a system of checks and balances. Every so often check on how you're doing and balance out any problems you find.

- Rely on thin habits.

  Every now and then read over thin habits to refresh your resolve to eat well.
- Eat commonsense portions.

  A commonsense amount of any food is a good choice.
- Use your Daily Food Diary.

  Once or twice a month, more often if you'd like, tally a day's intake to see if you're still in your target calorie zone.
- Use your Weekly Activity Log.

  Every so often track a week's activity to be sure you are still as active as you should be for good health and a healthy weight.
- Eat a calcium-rich diet—*calcium counts!*

  Adequate calcium keeps you healthy and helps you stay slim.
- Drink 8 to 10 glasses of water or other fluids each day— *water works!*

  Being well hydrated helps your body work better and burn calories more efficiently.
- When you need a hunger chaser—*use pectin!*

  Once in a while, around the holidays, or whenever you need a little help, go back to using your pectin hunger chaser to keep your appetite in check.
- Enjoy the adventure of eating.

  You won't stick with something you don't enjoy.

Appendix 1

Your Weekly Activity Goal

Everything counts—planned activities and real life fitness—walking, gardening, golf, tennis, even housework. The more activity, the more calories you burn. Activity builds muscles and muscles burn calories, 70 times faster than fat.

Activity gets you to your target weight faster. In Chapter 7, you set your activity goal. Depending on whether you are currently inactive, somewhat active or moderately active, you'll be aiming to use up 500 to 1000 calories a week. The ultimate goal is to double this amount as you become more fit.

Your activity goal is to burn _____ calories each week.

You'll keep track of your daily activity on your Weekly Activity Log, page 298. Every few weeks, as your fitness improves, increase your activity goal. If your initial goal is to burn 750 calories, aim for 1000 instead. You'll feel so good, losing weight and getting fit, that you'll look forward to the extra activity.

It's easy to keep track of the calories you burn. On the chart, Using Up Calories Through Activity, page 294, find the activity you've done and the weight column closest to your current weight. Multiply the calories burned in 1 minute by the number of minutes you were active. For example, if you weigh 150 pounds and you washed the kitchen floor for 15 minutes you used up 69 calories.

Housework (washing floors)

4.6 (calories burned in 1 minute) × 15 minutes = 69 calories

If you take a 30 minute leisurely walk, too, you'd burn 96 more calories.

Walking (2 miles per hour)

3.2 (calories burned in 1 minute) × 30 minutes = 96 calories

If your activity goal for the week is to burn 750 calories, you've already burned 165 through these 2 simple activities.

Keep track of the activity calories you burn each day as well as your total for the week. It's easy to reach your Weekly Activity Goal.

Using Up Calories Through Activity

Pounds: Activity	100	125	150 Calories Used Per Minute	175	200
Archery	3.1	4.0	4.8	5.6	6.4
Auto repair	2.8	3.5	4.2	4.8	5.5
Badminton	3.6	4.6	5.4	6.4	7.3
Baseball	3.1	4.0	4.7	5.5	6.3
Basketball	4.9	6.2	9.9	11.5	13.2
Bicycling					
5 mph	1.9	2.4	2.9	3.4	3.9
10 mph	4.2	5.3	6.4	7.4	8.5
Bowling	2.7	3.4	4.1	4.5	5.5
Boxing	6.2	7.8	9.3	10.9	12.4
Calisthenics, light	3.4	4.3	5.2	6.1	7.0
Canoeing					
4 mph	4.4	5.5	6.7	7.8	8.9
Carpentry	2.6	3.2	3.8	4.6	5.3
Chopping wood	4.8	6.0	7.2	8.4	9.6
Croquet	2.7	3.4	4.1	4.7	5.4

Activity	Pounds: 100	125	150	175	200
	Calories Used Per Minute				
Dancing					
Moderate (waltz)	3.1	4.0	4.8	5.6	6.4
Active (square, disco)	4.5	5.6	6.8	7.9	9.1
Aerobic dance	6.0	7.6	9.1	10.8	12.1
Fencing, moderately	3.3	4.1	5.0	5.8	6.7
Fishing	2.8	3.5	4.2	4.9	5.6
Football, touch	5.5	6.9	8.3	9.7	11.1
Gardening					
Lawn mowing, manual	3.0	3.8	4.6	5.2	5.9
Lawn mowing, power	2.7	3.4	4.1	4.7	5.4
Light gardening	2.4	3.0	3.6	4.2	4.8
Weeding	3.9	4.9	5.9	6.8	7.8
Golf					
Twosome (carry clubs)	3.6	4.6	5.4	6.4	7.3
Foursome (carry clubs)	2.7	3.4	4.1	4.5	5.4
Gymnastics	3.0	3.8	4.5	5.3	6.0
Handball	6.5	6.2	9.9	11.5	13.2
Hiking					
3 mph	4.5	5.5	6.8	7.9	9.1
Hockey, field	5.0	7.6	9.1	10.8	12.1
Hockey, ice	6.6	8.3	10.0	11.7	13.4
Horseback riding					
Walk	1.9	2.4	2.9	3.4	3.9
Trot	2.7	3.4	4.1	4.8	5.4
Gallop	5.7	7.2	8.7	10.1	11.6
Horseshoes	2.5	3.1	3.8	4.4	5.2
House painting	2.3	2.9	3.5	4.0	4.6
Housework					
Dusting	1.8	2.3	2.6	3.1	3.5
Making beds	2.6	3.2	3.8	4.6	5.3
Washing floors	3.0	3.8	4.6	5.3	6.1
Washing windows	2.8	3.5	4.2	4.8	5.5

(continued)

Using Up Calories Through Activity (cont.)

Activity	Pounds: 100	125	150	175	200
		Calories Used Per Minute			
Ice skating	4.2	5.2	6.4	7.4	8.5
Judo	8.5	10.6	12.8	14.9	17.1
Karate	8.5	10.6	12.8	14.9	17.1
Lacrosse	9.5	11.9	14.3	16.6	19.0
Motorcycling	2.4	3.0	3.6	4.2	4.8
Mountain climbing	6.5	8.2	9.8	11.5	13.1
Paddle ball	5.7	7.2	8.7	10.1	11.6
Pool (billiards)	1.5	1.9	2.2	2.6	3.0
Racquetball	6.5	8.1	9.8	11.4	13.0
Rollerblading					
9 mph	4.2	5.3	6.4	7.4	8.5
Rowing	3.4	4.2	5.0	5.9	6.7
Rowing machine	9.1	11.4	13.7	16.0	18.2
Running, steady rate					
5 mph	6.0	7.6	9.1	10.8	12.2
7 mph	9.7	12.1	14.6	17.1	19.5
Sailing, small boat	4.2	5.2	6.4	7.4	8.5
Shoveling snow	5.2	6.5	7.8	8.9	10.2
Skiing, cross country					
2.5 mph	5.0	6.2	7.5	8.8	10.0
4 mph	6.5	8.2	9.9	11.5	13.2
Skiing, alpine downhill	6.4	8.0	9.6	11.2	12.8
Skindiving, moderate activity	9.4	11.8	14.1	16.5	18.8
Soccer	5.9	7.4	8.9	10.3	11.8
Squash	6.7	8.4	10.1	11.8	13.5
Swimming					
Backstroke	2.5	3.1	3.8	4.4	5.1
Breaststroke	3.1	4.0	4.8	5.6	6.4
Front crawl	4.0	5.0	6.0	7.0	8.0
Table tennis	3.4	4.3	5.2	6.3	7.2
Tennis					
Singles	5.0	6.2	7.5	6.8	10.0
Doubles	3.4	4.3	5.2	6.1	7.0
Typing	1.5	1.9	2.3	2.7	3.1
Volleyball	2.9	3.6	4.4	5.1	5.9

Pounds:	100	125	150	175	200
Activity	Calories Used Per Minute				
Walking					
2 mph	2.1	2.6	3.2	3.7	4.3
4 mph	4.2	5.3	6.4	7.4	8.5
Water skiing	5.0	6.2	7.5	8.8	10.0
Weight training					
Free weight	3.9	4.9	5.9	6.8	7.8
Nautilus	4.2	5.3	6.3	7.4	8.4
Universal	5.3	6.6	8.0	9.3	10.6

Weekly Activity Log

Activity	Minutes Spent at Activity	Calories Used/ Minute/_____* Pounds	Total Calories Burned
MONDAY			
		Monday Total	_____
TUESDAY			
		Tuesday Total	_____
WEDNESDAY			
		Wednesday Total	_____
THURSDAY			
		Thursday Total	_____
FRIDAY			
		Friday Total	_____
SATURDAY			
		Saturday Total	_____
SUNDAY			
		Sunday Total	_____

WEEKLY ACTIVITY GOAL _____   WEEKLY TOTAL   _____
CALORIES USED UP BY EXERCISE

*The weight closest to your current weight.

Appendix 2

Getting Started: A Basic Strength Training and Stretching Program

Strength Training

Strength training is the most popular fitness activity in America today.

Your muscles are incredibly active. They are busy even when you sleep. The more muscle (lean body mass) you have, the more calories you burn. Regular strength training (lifting weights) burns calories and builds muscles. But, did you realize that it also helps to lower cholesterol, prevent diabetes, ease chronic back pain, improve mood, build bones, and relieve arthritis?

The American College of Sports Medicine recommends a strength training session 2 to 3 times a week with a day of rest in between. A full-body series of exercises should take at least 20 to 30 minutes to complete. Some people enjoy strength training daily and will work the upper body one day and the lower body the next. This allows some of the muscles a full day to rest, while the other muscles are working.

A typical full-body strength training program has 8 to 10 exercises that work all the body's major muscle groups—chest, shoulders, arms, back, abdomen, buttocks, hips, and legs. You can do these exercises with free weights, weight machines, exercise bands or water workouts. All work equally well when done regularly. Choose the type of strength training program you enjoy or vary your routine to stay motivated.

Strength training programs are made up of "sets" and "reps." For example, a biceps curl is called a "set." It is done for a number of "reps" or repetitions—the number of times you lift and lower the weight. Sets and reps can be done two ways—multiple sets or a single set. Multiple sets would be 3 sets of biceps curls for 10 repetitions each. Or you can do one set of biceps curls for 10 to 12 repetitions.

Fitness professionals continually debate which system is best, multiple sets or a single set of each major muscle group. To build larger muscles, multiple sets are probably the best route. But for general fitness and improved strength, research shows that one set per major body part works great.

Start with a weight that will challenge you but does not cause pain. You should be able to lift and lower the weight at least 8 times, with slightly increasing difficulty. You may feel muscle soreness after your initial workouts but you should never be in pain. Lift and lower slowly. Breathe out as you lift and breathe in as you lower. Breathing rhythmically is an important part of the exercise. When you can easily lift a weight for more than 15 reps you can progress to a heavier one. If you have never done strength training before, even lifting a 1 pound weight will improve strength and endurance. You decide where you should start. Set goals you can reach.

On the next few pages is a simple strength training program. It will work all major muscle groups beginning with the upper body and then the lower body. If you wish, you can divide the exercises into two parts to work half the body one day and the other half the next. If you are new to strength training or have not done it for a while, this program is a good place to start. To go further there are books, videos, fitness clubs, "Y"s and personal trainers to help you.

Upper Body

Biceps Curl

Strengthens your upper arm or biceps muscle.

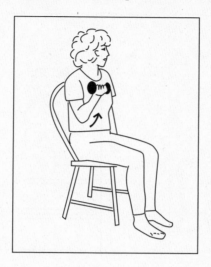

- Stand straight with feet flat on the floor, bend knees slightly.
- Hold weight at your side, arms straight and close to your body, palms in.
- Lift weights by bending elbows and rotating palms in to face shoulder.
- Lower slowly to starting position.
- Repeat 8 to 12 times.

This exercise can be done one arm at a time or both together. It can also be done sitting in an armless chair with back support.

Triceps Extension

Strengthens muscles in the back of the upper arm or triceps.

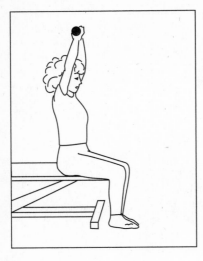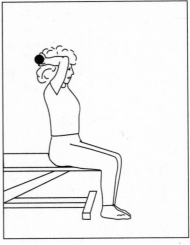

- Grasp a weight, with each hand on one end of the ball shape, palms forward.
- Raise the weight straight over your head, keeping your elbows straight up and your upper arms close to your head.
- Lower the weight behind your head by bending your elbows and then raise the weight up again to the starting overhead position.
- Repeat 8 to 12 times.

This exercise can be done sitting on a bench or on the edge of a chair. You can also hold the weight in one hand and work one arm at a time.

Alternate Triceps Extension

Use this position if the shoulder joint is painful in the overhead position.

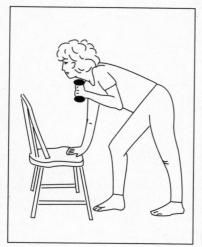 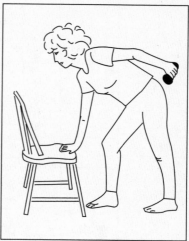

- Stand next to a chair seat.
- Lean forward at the waist, resting one hand on the chair seat.
- Hold the weight in your free hand, palm toward your body.
- Bend your elbow; keeping your arm close to your body, extend arm straight out behind you.
- Bring arm forward to bent elbow position.
- Repeat 8 to 12 times.
- Repeat with other arm.

Lateral Rise

Strengthens the shoulder muscles or deltoids.

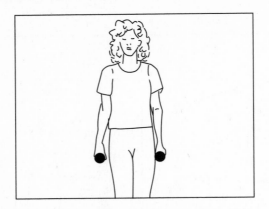

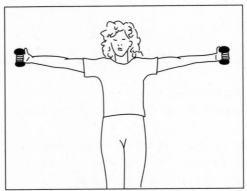

- Stand straight with your arms hanging straight down at your sides, palms facing in with a weight in each hand.
- Slowly raise weights, turning your palms to face forward with your thumbs pointing up; raise your arms up parallel to the floor (no higher).
- Lower arms to starting position.
- Repeat 8 to 12 times.

To start, you can do this exercise by lifting the weight up partially until you can comfortably lift the weights parallel to the floor.

Shoulder Shrug

Strengthens the shoulder and back muscles or trapezius.

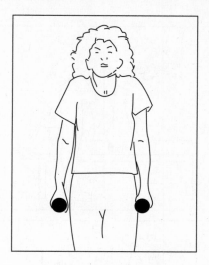

- Stand straight with your arms hanging straight down at your sides, palms toward the body with a weight in each hand.
- Keeping your arms straight, raise your shoulders as high as possible, pause and lower to the starting position.
- Repeat 8 to 12 times.

Dumbbell Row

Strengthens the back and upper arms or latissimus dorsi and biceps muscles.

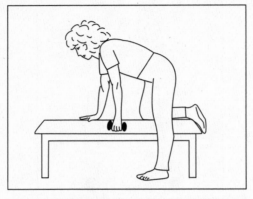

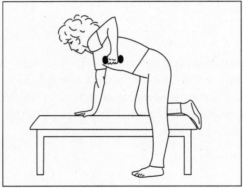

- Place one knee on a bench, bend over until your body is parallel to the floor, place your arm on the bench for support.
- With the free arm fully extended toward the floor, grip a weight in your hand, palm toward the bench, raise the weight up close to your body with a pulling motion, to the height of your waist.
- Extend your arm back down to the straight position.
- Repeat 8 to 12 times.
- Repeat exercise with other arm.

Flat Press

Strengthens the muscles of the chest or pectorals.

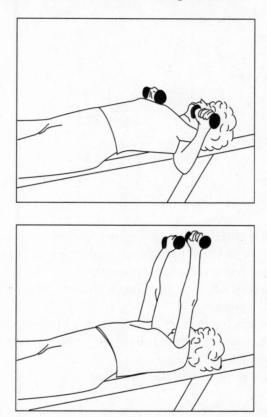

- Lie on a bench with a weight in each hand, palms facing forward and the inner edge of the weight touching your chest.
- Extend your arms up until they are straight, with the weights directly above your upper chest.
- Lower the weight to the starting position with the weight touching your chest and your elbows below the bench; this will give a full stretch to your chest muscles.
- Repeat 8 to 12 times.

Lower Body

Leg Extension

Strengthens the front thigh muscles or quadriceps.

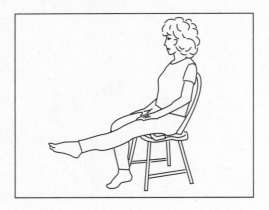

- Sit in a chair with back support and put a rolled-up towel under your knees to lift them slightly, so that only the balls of your feet and toes are on the floor.
- Place your hands on your thighs and you will feel your thigh muscles working.
- Raise one leg in front of you parallel to the floor, flex your foot to point your toes toward the ceiling. Lower the leg.
- Repeat 8 to 12 times.
- Repeat exercise with the other leg.

Ankle weights can be used to do this exercise. You can also do the exercise by alternating the legs for a set of 8 to 12 reps.

Leg Curl

Strengthens the muscles in back of the thigh or hamstrings.

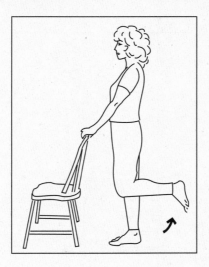

- Using a table or chair back for balance, stand straight with feet shoulder width apart.
- Bend your leg from the knee, keeping the upper leg still, and bringing your lower leg up and back as far as possible toward the thigh.
- Repeat 8 to 12 times.
- Repeat exercise with the other leg.

Ankle weights can be used to do this exercise. This exercise can also be done lying on your stomach on a mat. Bending from the knee, lift one leg at a time off the mat, up and back as far as possible toward the thigh.

Calf Raise

Strengthens the muscles in the ankles and back of the lower leg or the calf muscles.

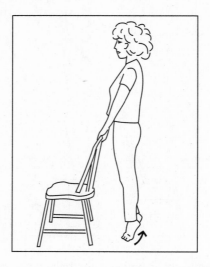

- Using a table or chair back for balance, stand straight with feet shoulder width apart.
- Slowly raise up on tiptoes, as high as possible, hold, and lower till feet are flat on the ground.
- Repeat 8 to 12 times.

Ankle weights can be used to do this exercise. You can also do this exercise standing on one leg with the nonsupporting leg bent up at the knee. As balance gets better, you can do this exercise without a support.

Leg Extension

Strengthens muscles in the hips and buttocks or gluteus maximus.

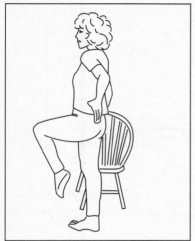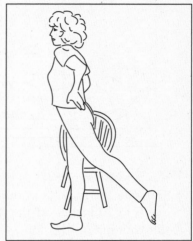

- Standing sideways, hold on to a chair for support.
- Bending at the knee, raise your outside leg till the ankle of that leg is as high as the knee of the stationary (straight, inside) leg.
- Simultaneously lower and extend back your raised leg until it is behind you and your knee is almost straight.
- Keep your upper body as still as possible, letting your buttocks muscles do the work.
- Without placing your working leg on the floor, repeat the exercise 8 to 12 times.
- Switch to the other leg and repeat the set.

Ankle weights can be used to do this exercise.

Alternate Leg Extension

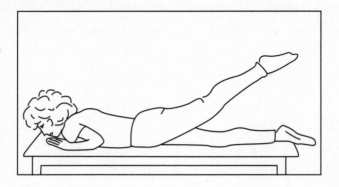

- Lie on your stomach.
- Tighten the muscles in the front of the thigh and lift your leg 8 to 10 inches off the floor; do not bend your knee or lift your hip off the floor.
- Lower leg to the floor.
- Repeat 8 to 12 times.
- Repeat with other leg.

Ankle weights can be used to do this exercise.

Chair Stand

Strengthens muscles in the stomach and thighs or the abdominals and quadriceps.

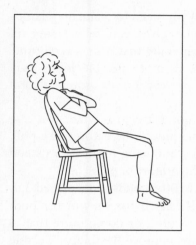

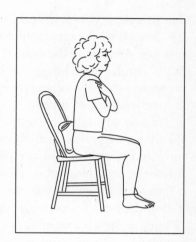

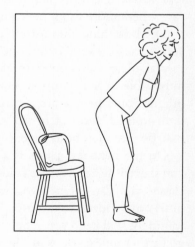

- Using a chair with a straight back, sit in the middle to front of the seat, feet flat on the floor and arms crossed in front of your chest.
- Lean back against the chair in a half-reclining position.
- Without using your hands or arms, sit up straight and stand up slowly. Sit back down.
- Repeat 8 to 12 times.

This exercise can be done holding weights in your hands for more resistance.

Stretching

Stretching is one of the most powerful weapons against aging.

Ten minutes, 3 times a week, is all you need to maintain flexibility. Stretching loosens muscles and gives you fuller range of motion, preventing the natural tightening that occurs with time. With regular stretching, you'll have more flexible joints, will avoid muscle strains and tears, prevent muscle soreness, and reduce your risk of injury.

It's easy to stretch correctly. A good stretch is when you ease slowly into a position, reaching the point where you feel a pull, hold and release. A bad stretch is a bouncing motion to extend further or stretching till you feel discomfort or pain.

Stretches should be held for 10 to 30 seconds and repeated 3 to 4 times for each muscle group. Research has shown that both holding a stretch longer than 30 seconds or doing more than 4 repetitions of a movement does not improve flexibility. A classic case where more is not necessarily better.

The best thing about stretching is that it can be done anytime you want to take a 10-minute "time-out" break. It requires no special place or equipment, and if done correctly, it's almost impossible to hurt yourself. Don't measure your own progress by others. Some people are naturally loose-jointed while others are tight-jointed. Most of us fall somewhere in between. But everyone, despite their body type, can increase flexibility by stretching.

On the next few pages is a simple stretching program to get you started. When you are ready to go further there are stretching classes you can attend, yoga and tai chi programs to try, and instructive videos to explore. The basic stretching, when done routinely, will keep you supple and flexible, so there is no need to go further unless you want the added challenge.

Stretching Exercises

Hamstring Stretch

Stretches the muscles in the back of the thigh.

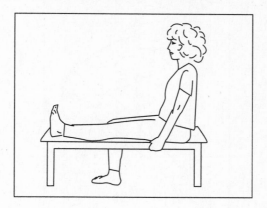

- Sit sideways on a bench, keeping one leg straight in front of you on the bench and the other foot flat on the floor next to the bench.
- Straighten your back and lean forward from the hips (not the waist) until you feel stretching in the back of the leg on the bench.
- Hold 10 to 30 seconds, release.
- Repeat 3 to 4 times.
- Switch to other leg and repeat.

Alternate Hamstring Stretch

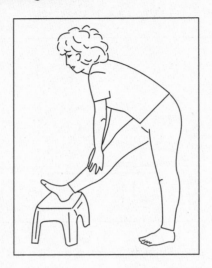

- Stand in front of a low stool or staircase.
- Place the heel of one foot on a step, toes up.
- Lean forward until you feel stretching in the back of the leg on the step.
- Hold 10 to 30 seconds, release.
- Repeat 3 to 4 times.
- Repeat with other leg.

Calf Stretch

Stretches the lower back leg muscles.

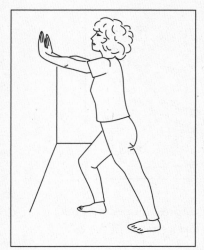 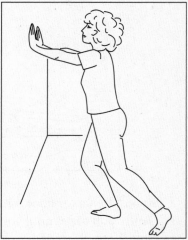

- Stand with arms at shoulder height and place hands flat against a wall.
- Step back 1 to 2 feet with the right leg, keeping both feet flat on the floor.
- Bend the left knee. You should feel a stretch in the right calf. If not, step back farther on the right leg.
- Hold 10 to 30 seconds, release.
- Repeat 3 to 4 times.
- Repeat on other leg.

Alternate Calf Stretch

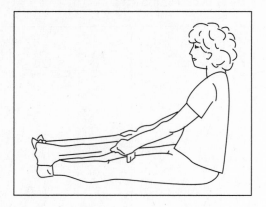

- Sit on a bench or floor with a towel looped around a foot.
- Gently pull towel until you feel a stretch in the calf.
- Hold 10 to 30 seconds, release.
- Repeat 3 to 4 times.
- Repeat on other leg.

Ankle Stretch

Stretches front ankle muscles.

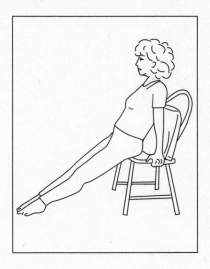

- Sit at the edge of a chair stretching your legs out in front of you, heels on the floor.
- Bend your ankles toward you and hold; then bend your ankles away from you and hold.
- Repeat 3 to 4 times.

Triceps Stretch

Stretches the muscles in the back of the upper arm.

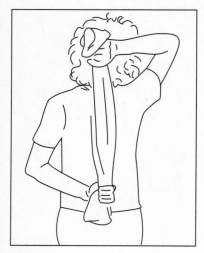 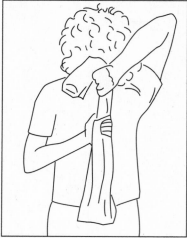

- Holding a towel in your right hand, raise your arm and bend your elbow so that the towel drapes down your back.
- Grab the bottom of the towel with your left hand using the left hand to climb up the towel as high as you can.
- As the left hand climbs up the towel the right arm will be pulled down.
- Repeat 3 to 4 times.
- Repeat with other arm.

The ultimate goal of this stretch is to have the two hands meet behind your back. Stretch as close as you can comfortably.

Wrist Stretch

Stretches the muscles in the wrists and upper arms.

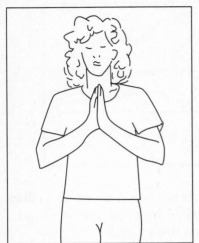 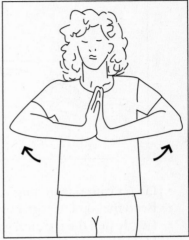

- Elbows down, place your hand in front of your chest in a praying position.
- Pressing your hands together, raise elbows until they are parallel to the floor.
- Hold 10 to 30 seconds, release.
- Repeat 3 to 4 times.

Quadriceps Stretch

Stretches the muscles in the front of thighs.

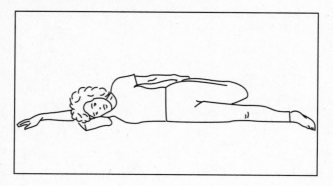

- Lie on your side, resting your head on your arm or a pillow.
- Bend the top knee, grabbing the foot with your top hand.
- Gently pull the leg until your thigh stretches.
- Hold 10 to 30 seconds, release.
- Repeat 3 to 4 times.

Repeat with other leg.

Double Hip Rotation
Stretches the outer muscles of the hips and thighs.

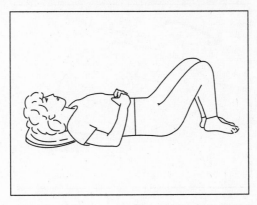

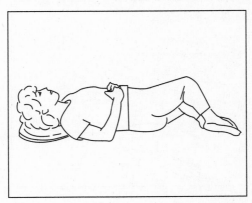

- Lie flat on the floor, knees bent.
- Keeping shoulders and back on the floor and knees together, lower both legs to one side.
- Hold 10 to 30 seconds, release to knees-up position.
- Repeat toward other side.
- Continue alternating sides 3 to 4 times.

This stretch can also be done as a single hip rotation, lowering one leg at a time. The single hip rotation stretches the pelvis and inner thigh muscles.

Shoulder Rotation

Stretches shoulder muscles.

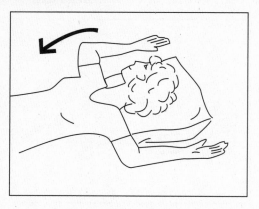

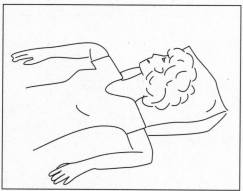

- Lie flat on the floor, legs out straight.
- With arms at shoulder height, bend elbows with palms up and hands pointing toward your head.
- Slowly raise bent arms up toward the ceiling and roll them forward toward your hips, keeping arms bent.
- Reverse the movement until the arms are flat on the floor alongside your head.
- Repeat 3 to 4 times.

Do not do this exercise if you feel a pain or sharp pinching sensation in the shoulder.

Neck Rotation
Stretches the neck muscles.

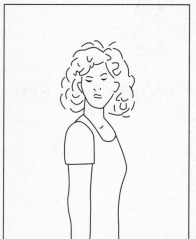 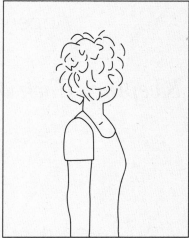

- Stand or sit up straight.
- Slowly turn your head to one side, hold 10 to 30 seconds. Slowly turn to the opposite side and hold.
- Repeat each side 3 to 4 times.

Getting Started: The American College of Sports Medicine recommends:

Strength Training: 3 to 5 times a week—20 to 60 minutes a session.

Stretching: 2 to 3 times a week—10 to 30 minutes a session

Appendix 3

Keeping Track of What You Eat

On average, people cut calories by 10% when they keep track of what they eat. 30% to 50% of those who kept a food record changed their eating habits. A food diary is the most important tool a dieter can use for food awareness.

"What have you eaten today?" is one of the first questions we ask. Some people can't remember what they've had for breakfast, they pay so little attention to eating. Others have no idea how much they ate. Few can accurately estimate portion sizes or calories.

We know it's a chore to write down everything you eat and keep track of the calories, but it's worth it. "After a week of writing down calories, most people have a good idea how many calories are in about 75% of what they eat." says Daniel S. Kirschenbaum, professor of psychiatry and behavioral science at Northwestern Medical School in Chicago. His research team found that people who kept a daily record of what they ate lost weight and kept it off, even losing during the difficult holiday season between Thanksgiving and Christmas.

Keeping a daily food diary works. It makes your efforts real, offers a continual reinforcement of your goal, and puts the responsibility for making food choices squarely on you. You are in control. You make choices. You write down those choices. If you are honest with yourself, you have, right there in front of you, an immediate assessment of how you're doing. Made the right choices? Great! Keep up the good work. Made choices that might derail your dieting goals? Relax! Your whole diet plan won't be ruined by one meal or snack. Use your food diary to put your eating plan back on track with your next meal or snack.

Many of our clients balk at the idea of having to write down everything they eat every day. We appreciate that this is a big job. We strongly recommend that as you start *Get Skinny the Smart Way* you write down everything you eat for the first week. After that you can keep track every other day or just a few days a week, to be sure you stay on target. Some people get so used to keeping a food diary and it becomes such a useful tool, they enjoy doing it daily. Others fall back on the tool during more stressful times, like holidays, vacations, business trips. Knowing the importance of a food diary and how to use it can be a great ally in achieving your weight loss goal. Use it to your advantage.

Keeping Track

Your Daily Food Diary not only gives you a place to record what you've eaten, but it will tell you a lot about your eating habits as well. No one will ever see what you write down, so there is no advantage to cheating. Be honest and you may find out a lot about how you eat, why you eat and what you eat.

Why is the day of the week important? Some days of the week can be trigger days that cause us to eat differently or more than usual. Saturday and Sunday are often considered atypical days. You may go out more. You may be home and have greater access to food and snacks. Some people eat more on Friday, celebrating the end of a work week. Some eat more on Monday to reduce the stress of a new week. As you record your daily intake, you will discover your own eating pattern. If some days trigger overeating and you are aware of this, it will be easier to change the pattern.

The Daily Food Diary is set up in three time periods throughout the day. We appreciate that many of us eat on a crazy schedule. Three meals a day is anything but typical for many of our clients. Breaking the day into three periods is an easier way to keep track of how you eat. It will also show you when you do most of your eating. Ideally, the best way to eat is to get most of your calories early in the day, providing ample time to use them up through activity. For most of us, this is the reverse of what we do. We may skip breakfast, eat a light lunch and then have a large evening meal and snack after dinner. Your goal will be to spread your meals and snacks out more evenly throughout the day. Recording when you eat will help you accomplish this.

A.M. is any time from midnight till noon. Many people eat late at night or even in the middle of the night. This is often a way to cope with stress or anxiety. If you do this regularly, you'll need to work on reducing your stress. Middle-of-the-night noshing results in calories that are rarely needed and hard to work off. A.M. eating will include eating during the night, breakfast, and any morning snack, like an A.M. coffee break.

SMART STUFF

A study conducted at St. Luke's-Roosevelt Obesity Research Center in New York City showed that men are more likely than women to eat late at night or during the night. Some ate up to 70% of their calories at night, often picking foods high in fat, sugar and salt.

Midday is any time from noon until dinner. For most this will include lunch and any afternoon or pre-dinner snack.

P.M. is dinnertime through midnight. It will include your evening meal, and after dinner, TV or bedtime snacks.

Next you'll record the portion size of every food you eat. In Chapter 6 you read about commonsense portions and visual clues you can use to estimate portion sizes. Do your best to stick to these realistic food portions. *Eating commonsense portions* is a thin habit.

Starting on page 332 is a list of the calories in over 600 foods. This will help you to record the amount of calories in each food you eat so that you stay within the target calorie zone you set for yourself in Chapter 7. If you would like a bigger calorie counter we can recommend two other resources we've written, *The Calorie Counter* and *The Most Complete Food Counter*. Both list the calories for over 20,000 foods.

By subtotaling your calories three times during the day, you can make adjustments. This is also a way to balance unexpected situations. For example, knowing you have to attend an afternoon reception for work, you can skip your usual coffee break and plan a lighter lunch to compensate for the extra calories eaten at the reception.

Why does it matter if you eat alone or with company? Because many of us eat differently in private. You may begin to see a pattern of how you handle food when you are alone compared to eating with someone. Some people eat more when they eat alone. Others eat more when they linger over food with company. Learning this about yourself will help you eat commonsense portions in most situations.

And finally, we want you to use *Get Skinny*'s powerful dieting aids every day. The pectin hunger chaser makes you feel fuller longer, and reduces your desire to overeat. By eating at least 2 excellent sources of calcium and taking a 600 milligram calcium supplement, you'll lose rather than store extra body fat. And be sure you get at least 8 cups of water or other fluids each day. Water is a powerful calorie burner. Until it becomes a habit, keeping track of your daily dieting aids will help you lose weight faster.

Daily Food Diary

Your Target Calorie Zone _____

Day _____   Date _____

FOOD	PORTION	CALORIES	ATE ALONE	WITH COMPANY

A.M.

A.M. Calorie Total _____

Midday

Midday Calorie Total _____

P.M.

P.M. Calorie Total _____

Day's Calorie Total _____

Did You Have?

Pectin Hunger Chaser	2 Excellent Calcium Sources	Water and Other Fluids 8 cups a day
___ Yes ___ No	1___ 2___ + 600 mg supplement ___	_ _ _ _ _ _ _ _ (1 cup = 8 ounces)

Abbreviations

diam = diameter
fl = fluid
g = gram
in = inch
lbs = pounds
lg = large
med = medium
oz = ounce
pkg = package
reg = regular
serv = serving
sm = small
sq = square
tbsp = tablespoon
tsp = teaspoon
w/ = with
w/o = without

Note

In the following table, brand names are set Upper and Lowercase; recipes found elsewhere in this book are set in *Upper and Lowercase Italics.*

Food	Portion	Calories
ABALONE		
cooked	4 oz	119
ALFALFA		
sprouts	1 tbsp	1
ALMONDS		
oil roasted salted	1 oz	174
ANCHOVY		
fillet	1	8
paste	1 tsp	14
APPLE		
applesauce	½ cup	97
Baked Apple	1	143
fresh	1	81
juice	1 cup	116
APRICOTS		
dried halves	5	42
fresh	3	51
nectar	1 cup	141
ARTICHOKE		
fresh	1 med (4 oz)	60
hearts cooked	½ cup	42
ARUGULA		
raw	½ cup	2
ASPARAGUS		
canned	1 cup	40
cooked	4 spears	14
AVOCADO		
fresh	1	324
BACON		
fried	3 strips	109
substitute cooked	1 strip	25
BAGEL		
mini	1 (1 oz)	100
plain toasted	1 (3½ in) 2 oz	195
BANANA		
fresh	1	105
BASS		
sea cooked	4 oz	140
striped cooked	4 oz	140
BEANS		
baked beans	½ cup	161
Mustard Pepper Beans	1 cup	212
Refried Bean Wrap	1 wrap	185
refried beans	½ cup	43
Southwestern Chili Stew with Polenta	1 serv	182

Food	Portion	Calories
BEANS		
Spicy Rice & Beans	1 cup	170
sprouts	½ cup	8
vegetarian baked beans	½ cup	140
BEEF		
brisket braised	4 oz	280
corned beef hash reduced fat	½ cup	140
flank steak braised	4 oz	299
ground extra lean broiled	4 oz	289
ground regular broiled	4 oz	328
london broil	4 oz	240
porterhouse steak broiled	4 oz	347
prime rib roasted	4 oz	425
roast beef deli sliced	2 oz	140
shortribs braised	4 oz	337
sirloin broiled	4 oz	305
Slow-Cooked Barbecue Beef	1 serv	242
t-bone steak broiled	4 oz	292
tenderloin cooked	4 oz	258
top round broiled	4 oz	253
BEETS		
sliced cooked	1 cup	76
BISCUIT		
plain	1 (2 oz)	212
w/egg	1 (4.8 oz)	316
w/egg & ham	1 (6.7 oz)	442
BLACK BEANS		
cooked	1 cup	227
BLACKEYE PEAS		
cooked	1 cup	198
BLUEBERRIES		
fresh	1 cup	82
BLUEFISH		
fresh baked	4 oz	180
BRAN		
Kretschmer Toasted Wheat Bran	⅓ cup	57
Quaker Oat Bran	¼ cup	75
BRAZIL NUTS		
dried	1 oz	186
BREAD		
banana	1 slice (2 oz)	195
challah egg bread	1 slice (1.4 oz)	115
focaccia rosemary	1 piece (3.5 oz)	251
french	1 slice (1 oz)	78
italian	1 slice (1 oz)	81
pita	1 reg (2 oz)	165
pita	1 sm (1 oz)	78
raisin	1 slice	71

Food	Portion	Calories
BREAD		
rye	1 slice	83
seven grain	1 slice	70
white toasted	1 slice	80
whole wheat	1 slice	90
wrap	1 (6 in) 1 oz	100
BREADCRUMBS		
seasoned	1 tbsp	50
seasoned	¼ cup	200
BREADSTICKS		
sesame	2	100
wheat	2	80
BROCCOLI		
spears cooked	1 cup	50
BROWNIE		
plain	1 (2 in sq) 2.1 oz	243
BRUSSELS SPROUTS		
cooked	1 cup	60
BUCKWHEAT GROATS		
groats cooked	1 cup	182
Kasha Delight	1 cup	159
BULGUR		
cooked	1 cup	151
Mediterranean Bulgur Salad	1 cup	87
BUTTER		
stick	1 tbsp	102
whipped	1 tbsp	80
CABBAGE		
green raw shredded	½ cup	9
green shredded cooked	½ cup	17
red raw shredded	½ cup	10
red shredded cooked	½ cup	16
CAKE		
angelfood	1 slice (1 oz)	73
carrot w/icing	¹⁄₁₂ cake (3.9 oz)	484
cheesecake	⅙ cake (2.8 oz)	256
coffeecake crumb topped	¹⁄₁₂ cake (2.1 oz)	240
eclair	1 (3 oz)	262
Pop-Tart Strawberry	1 (1.8 oz)	200
pound fat free	1 slice (1 oz)	80
CANADIAN BACON		
grilled	1 slice (0.75 oz)	32
CANDY		
butterscotch	1 piece (6 g)	24
caramels	1 piece (8 g)	31
milk chocolate	1 bar (1.55 oz)	226

Food	Portion	Calories
CANTALOUPE		
fresh	¼	47
CARROTS		
baby	1 cup	53
juice	6 oz	73
raw	1 (2.5 oz)	31
CASHEWS		
cashew butter	1 tbsp	94
dry roasted salted	1 oz	163
CAULIFLOWER		
cooked	1 cup	28
flowerets raw	3	14
CELERY		
raw	1 stalk (1.3 oz)	6
sticks	1 cup	12
CEREAL		
Apple Jacks	1 cup	110
Cheerios	1 cup	110
Cinnamon Mini Buns	1 cup	120
Cocoa Puffs	1 cup (1 oz)	120
Corn Chex	1 cup (1 oz)	110
corn grits yellow or white regular & quick as prep	1 cup	145
farina as prep	1 cup	117
Froot Loops	1 cup	120
Kix	1 cup	90
Lucky Charms	1 cup	120
oatmeal instant as prep	1 cup	138
Product 19	1 cup	100
puffed rice	1 cup	56
Rice Krispies	1 cup	88
Shredded Mini Wheats	1 cup	107
Special K	1 cup	110
Wheaties	1 cup	110
CEREAL BARS		
Rice Krispies Treats	1 (0.8 oz)	90
CHEESE		
american	2 oz	164
blue	2 oz	200
cheddar	2 oz	228
cheddar lowfat	2 oz	98
cheddar shredded	1 tbsp	25
mozzarella part skim	2 oz	144
muenster	2 oz	208
parmesan grated	1 tbsp	23
provolone	2 oz	200
ricotta fat free	½ cup	100
swiss	2 oz	214

Food	Portion	Calories
CHERRIES		
fresh	10	49
CHESTNUTS		
roasted	2 to 3 (1 oz)	70
CHICKEN		
boneless breaded & fried w/barbecue sauce	6 pieces (4.6 oz)	330
breast batter dipped & fried	½ breast (4.9 oz)	364
breast w/skin roasted	½ breast (3.4 oz)	193
breast w/o skin roasted	½ breast (3 oz)	142
broiler/fryer w/skin roasted	½ chicken (10.5 oz)	715
canned	4 oz	160
Chicken in Mushroom Gravy	1 serv	125
cornish hen w/skin roasted	½ hen (4 oz)	296
Curried Chicken & Vegetables	1 serv	273
drumstick w/skin batter dipped & fried	1 (2.6 oz)	193
drumstick w/skin roasted	1 (1.8 oz)	112
Mustard Chicken Breast	1 breast	197
ready-to-eat chicken sliced	4 oz	133
Slow-Cooked Hawaiian Chicken	1 serv	180
thigh w/skin roasted	1 (2.2 oz)	153
wing w/skin batter dipped & fried	1 (1.7 oz)	159
wing w/skin roasted	1 (1.2 oz)	99
CHICKPEAS		
cooked	1 cup	269
CHICORY		
raw	1 cup	16
CHIPS		
baked potato chips	1 oz	110
corn chips	1 oz	153
potato chips	1 oz	152
potato sticks	½ cup (0.6 oz)	94
tortilla chips	1 oz	140
CHOCOLATE		
chips semisweet	60 pieces (1 oz)	136
Chocolate Slush	1 serv	180
syrup	2 tbsp	82
CINNAMON		
cinnamon sugar	¼ tsp	6
ground cinnamon	1 tsp	6
CLAMS		
meat only	½ cup	118
meat only	4 oz	168
COCOA		
hot cocoa	1 cup	218
hot cocoa light	1 cup (6 oz)	93

Food	Portion	Calories
COCONUT		
fresh	1 piece (1 oz)	119
COD		
cooked	4 oz	119
Fisherman's Stew	1 serv	237
COFFEE		
cappuccino	1 cup (8 fl oz)	77
coffee con leche	1 cup (8 fl oz)	77
decaffeinated	6 oz	4
espresso	1 cup (3 fl oz)	2
latte w/skim milk	13 oz	88
latte w/whole milk	13 oz	152
regular	6 oz	4
whitener powder nondairy	1 tsp	11
COLESLAW		
mix w/o dressing	1 cup	16
COLLARDS		
cooked	1 cup	34
COOKIES		
animal crackers	10	110
Fig Newtons	1 (0.56 oz)	56
fortune	1 (0.28 oz)	30
graham	1 sq (0.24 oz)	30
meringue	1	25
CORN		
cooked	1 cup	120
cream style	1 cup	186
fritters	1 (1 oz)	62
on-the-cob	1 ear 6-inch	150
Salsa Corn Salad	1 cup	71
COTTAGE CHEESE		
creamed	½ cup	109
lowfat 1%	½ cup	82
nonfat	½ cup	80
Tangy Cottage Cheese Salad	1 serv	346
COUSCOUS		
Confetti Couscous	1 cup	173
cooked	1 cup (5.5 oz)	176
Couscous Tuna Salad	1 cup	173
CRAB		
cake	1 (2 oz)	160
soft-shell fried	1 (4.4 oz)	334
steamed meat only	4 oz	131
CRACKERS		
cheese	14 (0.5 oz)	71
melba toast	1 (5 g)	19
oyster cracker	1 (1 g)	4
saltines	1 (3 g)	13
whole wheat	1 (4 g)	18

Food	Portion	Calories
CRANBERRY		
juice cocktail	1 cup	147
wholeberry sauce	2 tbsp	50
CREAM		
half & half	1 tbsp	40
light coffee	1 tbsp	30
whipped	¼ cup	103
CREAM CHEESE		
regular	2 tbsp (1 oz)	100
soft light	2 tbsp (1.1 oz)	70
whipped	2 tbsp	70
CROISSANT		
plain	1 (2 oz)	232
CUCUMBER		
Balsamic Cucumber Salad	1 cup	50
fresh	1 (11 oz)	38
Greek Cucumber Salad	1 cup	72
kimchee	1 cup	72
spears	1 cup	14
CUSTARD		
baked	½ cup (5 oz)	148
DANISH PASTRY		
cheese	1 (3.2 oz)	353
fruit	1 (3.3 oz)	335
DATES		
whole dried	4	114
DELI MEATS/COLD CUTS		
bologna beef	1 oz	88
liverwurst pork	1 oz	92
salami cooked	1 oz	71
DOUGHNUTS		
glazed	1 (2.1 oz)	242
EGG		
deviled	2 halves	145
hard cooked	1	77
salad	½ cup	307
scrambled plain	1	100
sunny side up	1	91
EGGNOG		
eggnog	1 cup	342
EGGPLANT		
cooked	1 cup	26
ENDIVE		
chopped	1 cup	8

Food	Portion	Calories
ENGLISH MUFFIN		
plain	1	135
w/butter	1 (2.2 oz)	189
whole wheat	1	134
FAT		
lard	1 tbsp	115
shortening	1 tbsp	113
FIGS		
dried	3	110
FISH		
gefilte fish	1 piece (1.5 oz)	35
sticks	1 stick (1 oz)	76
FLOUNDER		
cooked	4 oz	132
Horseradish Crusted Flounder	1 serv (4 oz)	180
FRENCH TOAST		
slice frozen	1 slice	126
FRUIT		
fruit punch	8 oz	116
fruit salad	1 cup	79
snack pack mixed fruit	1 pkg (4 oz)	90
GELATIN		
all flavors	½ cup	128
low calorie	½ cup	8
GOAT		
roasted	4 oz	163
GRAPEFRUIT		
Glazed Pink Grapefruit	½	51
juice	1 cup	102
pink	½	37
red sections	1 cup	69
white sections	1 cup	76
GRAPES		
fresh	1 cup	55
fresh	10	36
juice	1 cup	155
GREEN BEANS		
canned	1 cup	60
fresh cooked	1 cup	44
italian	1 cup	70
raw	1 cup	34
HADDOCK		
cooked	4 oz	127
HALIBUT		
cooked	4 oz	159

Food	Portion	Calories
HAM		
canned extra lean roasted	4 oz	155
center slice lean roasted	4 oz	220
patty cooked	1 patty (2 oz)	203
salad	½ cup	287
sliced extra lean	1 oz	74
HAMBURGER		
double patty w/bun	1 reg	544
single patty w/bun	1 reg	275
single patty w/cheese & bun	1 reg	320
HEARTS OF PALM		
canned	1 (1.2 oz)	9
HERRING		
cooked	4 oz	229
pickled	1 oz	78
HONEY		
honey	1 tsp	21
HONEYDEW MELON		
cubed	1 cup	60
wedge	⅒ melon	46
HORSERADISH		
horseradish	1 tbsp	6
HOT DOG		
beef	1	150
beef low fat	1	100
corndog	1	460
turkey	1	102
HUMMUS		
hummus	¼ cup	112
ICE CREAM AND FROZEN DESSERTS		
Dixie Cup Chocolate	1 (3.5 fl oz)	125
Dixie Cup Strawberry	1 (3.5 fl oz)	112
Dixie Cup Vanilla	1 (3.5 fl oz)	116
vanilla	½ cup	178
vanilla light	½ cup	92
ICED TEA		
diet iced tea	10 oz	5
ICES AND ICE POPS		
fudgesicle	1 pop	60
italian ice	1 serv	75
Lemon Ice	½ cup	114
sorbet	½ cup	110
JAM/JELLY		
all fruit spread	1 tbsp	35
jam	1 tbsp (0.7 oz)	48
jelly	1 tbsp (0.7 oz)	52

Food	Portion	Calories
KALE		
fresh cooked	1 cup	42
KETCHUP		
ketchup	1 tbsp	16
KIDNEY BEANS		
canned	1 cup	208
KIWI		
kiwis	2	90
LAMB		
cubed lean only, broiled	4 oz	211
leg of Lamb roasted	4 oz	292
loin chop broiled	1 chop (2.3 oz)	201
rib chop broiled	4 oz	409
shank braised	4 oz	275
LEMONADE		
diet	12 oz	5
LENTILS		
cooked	1 cup	231
LETTUCE		
iceberg	1 leaf	3
iceberg shredded	1 cup	8
romaine shredded	1 cup	8
LIVER		
beef pan-fried	4 oz	245
chicken liver stewed	¾ cup (4 oz)	175
paté	2 tbsp (1 oz)	82
LOBSTER		
fresh cooked	4 oz	111
MACKEREL		
baked	4 oz	235
smoked	4 oz	338
MANGO		
fresh sliced	1 cup	100
MARGARINE		
stick	1 tbsp	100
whipped	1 tbsp	60
MARSHMALLOW		
marshmallow	1 reg (0.3 oz)	23
MATZO		
plain	1 (1 oz)	112
whole wheat	1 (1 oz)	99
MAYONNAISE		
regular	1 tbsp	110

Food	Portion	Calories
MILK		
1%	1 cup	102
2%	1 cup	121
buttermilk	1 cup	80
evaporated	½ cup	169
evaporated skim	½ cup	99
nonfat	1 cup	86
whole	1 cup	150
MILKSHAKE		
chocolate	1 (10 oz)	360
vanilla	1 (10 oz)	314
MILLET		
cooked	1 cup (6.1 oz)	207
MOLASSES		
molasses	1 tbsp (0.7 oz)	53
MUSHROOMS		
pieces	1 cup	38
whole	1 (0.4 oz)	3
MUSTARD		
mustard	1 tsp	5
NECTARINE		
fresh	1	67
NOODLES		
egg cooked	1 cup (5.6 oz)	213
rice noodles cooked	1 cup (6.2 oz)	192
OIL		
corn	1 tbsp	120
olive	1 tbsp	119
OKRA		
sliced cooked	8 pods	27
OLIVES		
ripe	1 sm	4
ONION		
chopped cooked	1 cup	94
fresh	1 med	60
Golden Onions & Mushrooms	1 cup	40
rings	2 (0.7 oz)	81
scallions	1 tbsp	2
ORANGE		
juice	1 cup	110
mandarin orange sections	1 cup	140
navel	1	65
sections	1 cup	85
OYSTERS		
battered & fried	6 (4.9 oz)	368
cooked	16 med (4 oz)	156

Food	Portion	Calories
PANCAKE/WAFFLE SYRUP		
low calorie	1 tbsp	12
maple	1 tbsp (0.8 oz)	52
pancake syrup	1 tbsp (0.7 oz)	57
PANCAKES		
plain	1 lg (6 in)	150
w/butter & syrup	2 (8.1 oz)	520
PAPAYA		
fresh sliced	1 cup	54
nectar	1 cup	142
PARSNIPS		
fresh cooked	1 cup	126
PASTA		
elbows cooked	1 cup (4.9 oz)	197
lasagna	1 piece (2.5 in × 2.5 in)	374
macaroni & cheese	2 cups	640
spaghetti cooked	1 cup (4.9 oz)	197
spaghetti w/meatballs & cheese	2 cups	814
vegetable pasta cooked	1 cup (4.7 oz)	172
whole wheat cooked	1 cup (4.9 oz)	174
PEACH		
fresh	1	37
Peach Sundae	1 serv	219
snack pack sliced in light syrup	1 pkg (4 oz)	60
PEANUT BUTTER		
chunky or smooth	2 tbsp	190
PEANUTS		
chocolate coated	10 (1.4 oz)	208
dry roasted	1 oz	164
mixed nuts salted	1 oz	169
Planters Reduced Fat Honey Roasted	⅓ cup (1 oz)	130
PEAR		
fresh	1	98
halves in light syrup	1 half	45
PEAS		
green cooked	1 cup	134
green raw	1 cup	116
peapods cooked	1 cup	30
PECANS		
dry roasted	1 oz	187
PEPPERS		
diced cooked	1 cup	26
green	1 (2.6 oz)	20
jalapeno	1 (0.5 oz)	4
red	1 (2.6 oz)	20
yellow	10 strips	14

Food	Portion	Calories
PERSIMMONS		
fresh	1	118
PICKLES		
dill	1 lg	20
sweet	1 (1.2 oz)	41
PIE		
apple	⅛ of 9 in pie (5.4 oz)	411
blueberry	⅛ of 9 in pie (5.2 oz)	360
cherry	⅛ of 9 in pie (6.3 oz)	486
lemon meringue	⅛ of 9 in pie (4.5 oz)	362
pecan	⅙ of 8 in pie (4 oz)	452
pumpkin	⅙ of 8 in pie (3.8 oz)	229
PIKE		
cooked	4 oz	128
PINEAPPLE		
fresh chunks	1 cup	100
fresh slice	1 slice	42
Glazed Pineapple	2 slices	135
juice	1 cup	139
Pineapple Slush Cocktail	1 cup	76
slices in light syrup	1 slice	30
PINK BEANS		
cooked	1 cup	252
PINTO BEANS		
cooked	1 cup	186
PISTACHIOS		
dried	1 oz	164
PIZZA		
cheese	1 slice (4 oz)	300
english muffin pizza w/mushrooms	2 halves	225
pepperoni	1 slice (4 oz)	320
PLANTAINS		
sliced cooked	1 cup	178
PLUMS		
fresh	1	36
POLLACK		
baked	4 oz	125
POPCORN		
air popped	2 cups	62
Mother's Popcorn Cake	1 (0.3 oz)	35
oil popped	2 cups	110
POPOVER		
popover	1 (1.4 oz)	90

Food	Portion	Calories
PORK		
center loin roast	4 oz	225
center loin chop cooked	4 oz	229
center rib chop cooked	4 oz	284
ribs country style braised	4 oz	336
tenderloin roasted	4 oz	185
POTATO		
baked topped w/cheese sauce	1	475
baked topped w/sour cream & chives	1	394
baked w/skin	1 med (6 oz)	200
boiled	1 cup	136
french fries take-out	1 reg (4 oz)	498
mashed	1 cup	222
Oven Roasted Fries	10 pieces (1 cup)	150
Oven Roasted Seasoned Red Potatoes	1 cup	150
potato salad	½ cup	179
PRETZELS		
chocolate covered	1 (0.4 oz)	50
whole wheat	2 sm (1 oz)	103
sticks	30	60
PRUNE		
dried	5	100
juice	1 cup	181
PUDDING		
bread pudding	½ cup (4.4 oz)	212
Old-Fashioned Rice Pudding	½ cup	157
Snack Pack Chocolate	1 pkg (4 oz)	170
Snack Pack Reduced Calorie Chocolate	1 pkg (4 oz)	100
Snack Pack Reduced Calorie Vanilla	1 pkg (4 oz)	100
Snack Pack Vanilla	1 pkg (4 oz)	170
tapioca	½ cup (5.3 oz)	189
RADICCHIO		
raw shredded	1 cup	10
RADISHES		
red raw	10	7
RAISINS		
golden	1 tbsp	27
seedless	¼ cup	109
RASPBERRIES		
fresh sliced	1 cup	61
RED BEANS		
canned	1 cup (4.6 oz)	180
RICE		
brown cooked	1 cup (6.8 oz)	216
Brown Rice Risotto	1 cup	179

Food	Portion	Calories
RICE		
cake	1 (0.3 oz)	35
glutinous cooked	1 cup (6.1 oz)	169
instant brown cooked	1 cup	170
instant white cooked	1 cup (5.8 oz)	162
Spicy Rice and Beans	1 cup	170
white cooked	1 cup	205
ROLL		
brown & serve	1 (1 oz)	85
hamburger whole wheat	1	110
hard	1 (3.5 in)	167
whole wheat	1 (1 oz)	75
RUTABAGA		
cooked mashed	1 cup	82
SALAD		
tossed w/o dressing	2 cups	100
SALAD DRESSING		
french	2 tbsp (1 oz)	160
french fat free	2 tbsp	45
italian	2 tbsp (1 oz)	110
italian fat free	2 tbsp (1 oz)	20
ranch fat free	2 tbsp	45
thousand island fat free	2 tbsp	40
SALMON		
baked	4 oz	213
cake	1 (4 oz)	321
canned	4 oz	157
lox (smoked)	2 oz	66
SALSA		
salsa	2 tbsp	10
SANDWICH		
Barbecue Chicken Sandwich	1	267
chicken fillet w/cheese lettuce mayonnaise & tomato	1	632
fish fillet w/tartar sauce	1	431
ham w/cheese	1	353
roast beef plain	1	346
roast beef w/cheese	1	402
steak w/tomato lettuce salt & mayonnaise	1	459
tuna salad submarine sandwich w/lettuce & oil	1	584
SARDINES		
canned in oil w/bone	2	50
canned in tomato sauce w/bone	1	68
SAUCE		
tartar sauce	2 tbsp	150
worcestershire	1 tbsp	6
Worcestershire Medley Pasta Sauce	1 serv	219

Food	Portion	Calories
SAUSAGE		
breakfast	1 link (0.5 oz)	48
Smothered Sausage & Onion	1 serv	219
turkey sausage	1 (2.5 oz)	126
SCALLOPS		
breaded & fried	5 (4 oz)	309
cooked	4 oz	100
Scallops in Wine Sauce	1 serv	126
SCROD		
baked	4 oz	119
SHELLFISH SUBSTITUTES		
crab or lobster substitute	1 oz	28
One-Dish Seafood Dinner	1 serv	164
SHERBET		
orange	½ cup (4 fl oz)	132
SHRIMP		
breaded & fried	6 to 8 (6 oz)	454
cooked	8 lg (2 oz)	60
SMOOTHIE		
Blueberry Pectin Smoothie	1 serv	226
Fruit Smoothie	1 serv	117
High Energy Drink	2 cups	234
SODA		
club	12 oz	0
cola	12 oz	151
diet cola	12 oz	2
ginger ale	12 oz	124
orange	12 oz	177
root beer	12 oz	152
SOLE		
cooked	4 oz	132
SOUP		
chicken broth	1 cup	15
chicken noodle	1 cup	75
corn & cheese chowder	1 cup	286
hot & sour	1 cup	99
onion soup gratinée	1 serv	492
Quick Pasta e Fagiole	2 cups	260
split pea w/ham	1 cup	189
tomato	1 cup	86
wonton	1 cup	205
SOUR CREAM		
fat free	2 tbsp	26
sour cream	2 tbsp	60
SOY		
High Energy Drink	2 cups	234
soy (garden) burger	1 (3 oz)	110

Food	Portion	Calories
SOY (cont.)		
soy milk	1 cup	79
soy sauce light or regular	1 tbsp	5
soybeans roasted & toasted	¼ cup	123
SPAGHETTI SAUCE		
alfredo	½ cup (4.4 oz)	360
basil pesto	¼ cup (2.2 oz)	320
marinara	½ cup (4.5 oz)	70
Savory Bolognese Pasta Sauce	1 cup	151
SPINACH		
cooked	1 cup	42
raw chopped	1 cup	12
SQUASH		
Quick-Baked Acorn Squash	1 cup	120
STRAWBERRIES		
fresh sliced	1 cup	45
STUFFING/DRESSING		
bread	½ cup	178
SUGAR		
brown	1 tsp	14
maple sugar candy	1 piece (1 oz)	100
powdered	1 tsp	10
white	1 tsp (4 g)	15
SUNFLOWER		
seeds salted	1 oz	175
SWEET POTATO		
baked w/skin	1 (4 oz)	135
candied	4 oz	165
TANGERINE		
fresh	1	37
TEA/HERBAL TEA		
brewed	6 oz	2
green tea	1 (6 oz) cup	0
herbal tea	1 (6 oz) cup	0
TOFU		
Ginger Tofu	1 serv (4 oz)	108
TOMATO		
canned seasoned diced	1 can (14 oz)	170
cherry tomatoes	1 cup	30
fresh	1 (4.5 oz)	26
juice	1 cup	43
Microwave Tomatoes	1 cup	30
stewed	1 cup	80
Tangy Tomato Salad	1 cup	49
TORTILLA		
corn	1 (6 in diam)	56
flour	1 (8 in diam) 1.2 oz	114

Food	Portion	Calories
TROUT		
baked	4 oz	216
TUNA		
canned in oil	4 oz	225
canned in water	4 oz	132
Couscous Tuna Salad	1 cup	173
tuna salad	1 cup	383
TURKEY		
breast w/skin roasted	4 oz	212
burger frozen as prep	1 (3 oz)	170
ground cooked	4 oz	251
leg w/skin roasted	1 (1.2 lbs)	1133
wing w/skin roasted	1 (6.5 oz)	426
TURNIPS		
cooked mashed	1 cup	94
greens cooked	1 cup	30
VEAL		
cutlet braised	4 oz	229
loin chop braised	1 chop (2.8 oz)	227
parmigiana	1 serv (8 oz)	531
sirloin w/bone roasted	4 oz	228
VEGETABLES		
mixed	1 cup	108
peas & carrots	1 cup	76
VINEGAR		
balsamic	1 tbsp	5
flavored	1 tbsp	2
WAFFLES		
toaster waffle	1 (4 in sq)	88
WALNUTS		
halves	¼ cup	190
WATER		
mineral water	1 cup	0
WATERMELON		
chunks	1 cup	51
wedge	¹⁄₁₆	152
WHEAT GERM		
wheat germ	2 tbsp	52
WHIPPED TOPPINGS		
nondairy pressurized	¼ cup	44
whipped topping	¼ cup	50
WHITEFISH		
smoked	2 oz	78
WHITING		
cooked	4 oz	131

Food	Portion	Calories
WILD RICE		
cooked	1 cup (5.7 oz)	166
WINE		
red	4 oz	88
white	4 oz	80
YOGURT		
nonfat flavored	8 oz	150
plain	8 oz	140
plain nonfat	8 oz	110
snack size flavored	4 oz	120
YOGURT FROZEN		
chocolate	½ cup	130
vanilla	½ cup	120
ZUCCHINI		
cooked	1 cup	28
Roasted Italian Zucchini Slices	3–4 slices	28

Resources

Allison, D.B., Fontaine, K.R., Manson, J.E., Stevens, J., and VanItally, T.B., Annual Deaths Attributable to Obesity in the United States, *Journal of the American Medical Association,* 282(16):1530, October 27, 1999.

American Cancer Society, Cancer Facts and Figures 2001. *American Journal of Public Health;* 88 (12):1814, 2001.

American College of Sports Medicine Position Stand, The Recommended Quantity and Quality of Exercise for Developing and Maintaining Cardiorespiratory and Muscular Fitness, and Flexibility in Healthy Adults, *Medicine & Science in Sports & Exercise,* 30(6):975, 1998.

Aronoff, N.J., Geliebter, A., and Zammit, G., Gender and Body Mass Index as Related to the Night-eating Syndrome in Obese Outpatients, *Journal of the American Dietetics Association,* 101(1):102, January 2001.

Berning, J.R. and Steen, S.N., *Nutrition for Sport & Exercise,* Aspen Publishers, Inc., Gaithersburg, MD, 1998.

Black, A.E. and Cole, T.J., Biased Over- or Underreporting Is Characteristic of Individuals Whether Over Time or by Different Assessment Methods, *Journal of the American Dietetics Association,* 101(1):70, January 2001.

Blumenthal, J.A., et. al, Effects of Exercise Training on Older Patients with Major Depression, *Archives of Internal Medicine,* 159: 2349, 1999.

Boyle, M.A. and Zyla, G., *Personal Nutrition,* 2nd Ed., West Publishing Company, St. Paul, MN, 1992.

Brown, C., Higgins, M., Donato, K., Rohde, F., Garrison, R., Obarzanek, E., Ernst, N., Horan, M., Body Mass Index and the Prevalence of Hypertension and Dyslipidemia, *Obesity Research,* 8(9):605, December 2000.

Brown, L.B. and Older, C. H-K., A Food Display Assignment and Handling Food Models Improves Accuracy of College Students' Estimates of Food Portions, *Journal of the American Dietetics Association,* 100(9):1053, September 2000.

Calle, E.E., Thun, M.J., Petrelli, J.M., Rodriquez, C., and Heath, C.W., Body Mass Index and Mortality in a Prospective Cohort of U.S. Adults, *The New England Journal of Medicine,* 341(15):1097, October 7, 1999.

Camelon, K.M., Hadell, K., Jamsen, P.T., Ketonen, K.J., Kohtamaki, H.M., Makimatilla, S., Tormala, M-L., and Valve, R.H., The Plate Model: A Visual Method of Teaching Meal Planning, *Journal of the American Dietetics Association,* 98(10):1155, October 1998.

Chambers, E., Godwin, S. and Vecchio, F., Strategies for Reporting Portion Sizes Using Dietary Recall Procedures, *Journal of the American Dietetics Association,* 100(8):891, August 2000.

Chocolate: Can It Be Part of Your Healthy Diet? *Vegetarian Nutrition & Health Letter,* 3(7):1, August 2000.

Clemens, L.H.E., Slawson, D.L. and Klesges, R.C., The Effect of Eating Out on Quality of Diet in Premenopausal Women, *Journal of the American Dietetics Association,* 99(4):442, April 1999.

Cordero-MacIntyre, Z., Lohnman, T. and Rosen, J., Weight Loss Is Correlated with an Improved Lipoprotein Profile in Obese Post-menopausal Women, *Journal of the American College of Nutrition,* 19(2):275, 2000.

Craig, M.R., Kristal, A.R., Cheney, C.L. and Shattuck, A.L., The Prevalence and Impact of "Atypical" Days in 4-day Food Records, *Journal of the American Dietetics Association,* 100(4):421, April 2000.

Crawford, S.L., A Longitudinal Study of Weight and the Menopause Transition, *Menopause,* 7: 96, March/April 2000.

Dulloo, A.G., Duret, C., Rohrer, D., Girandier, L., Mensi, N., Fathi, M., Chantre, P. and Vandermander, J., Efficacy of a Green Tea Extract Rich in Catechin Polyphenols and Caffeine in Increasing 24-H Energy Expenditure and Fat Oxidation in Humans, *American Journal of Clinical Nutrition,* 70(6):1040, June 1999.

Eckel, R.H. and Krauss, R.M., American Heart Association Call to Action: Obesity as a Major Risk Factor for Coronary Heart Disease, *Circulation,* 97:2099, 1998.

Exercise: A Guide from the National Institute on Aging, National Institutes of Health, National Institute on Aging, NIA Information Center, PO Box 8057, Gaithersburg, MD 20898–8057, Publication No. NIH 98–4258, 1998.

Expert Panel on the Identification, Evaluation, and Treatment of Overweight in Adults. *American Journal of Clinical Nutrition,* 68(4): 899, October 1998.

Fiatarone Singh, M.A., *Exercise, Nutrition and the Older Woman,* CRC Press, Boca Raton, FL, 2000.

Fogelholm, M., Kukkonem-Harjula, K, Nenonen, A. and Pasamen, M., Effects of Walking Training on Weight Maintenance After a Very-Low-Energy Diet in Premenopausal Obese Women, *Archives of Internal Medicine,* 160:2177, 2000.

Fulton, J.E., Masse, L.C., Tortolero, S.R., Watson, K.B., Heesch, K.C., Kohl III, H.W., Blair, S.N. and Caspersen, C.J., Field Evaluation of Energy Expenditure from Continuous and Intermittent Walking in Women, *Medicine & Science in Sports & Exercise,* 33(1): 163, 2001.

Fung, T.T., Rimm, E.B., Spiegelman, D., Rifai, N., Tofler, G.H., Willett, W.C. and Hu, F.B., Association between Dietary Patterns and Plasma Biomarkers of Obesity and Cardiovascular Disease Risk, *American Journal of Clinical Nutrition,* 73(1):61, January 2001.

Galuska, D.A., Will, J.C., Serdula, M.K. and Ford, E.S., Are Health Professionals Advising Obese Patients to Lose Weight?, *Journal of the American Medical Association,* 282(16):1576, October 27, 1999.

Georgiades, A., Sherwood, A., Elizabeth, C., Gullette, D., et al, Effects of Exercise and Weight Loss on Mental Stress-induced Cardiovascular Responses in Individuals with High Blood Pressure, *Hypertension,* 36:171, August 2000.

Grary, A.S. and Raab, C.A., On-line to Healthy Weights: Employed Women's Responses to Electronic Messages on Weight Management, *Journal of Nutrition Education,* 32(1):56, February 2000.

Hakim, A.A., Petrovitch, H., Burchfiel, C.M., et al., Effects of Walking on Mortality among Nonsmoking Retired Men, *New England Journal of Medicine,* 338(2):94, January 8, 1998.

Haller, C.A. and Benowitz, N.L., Adverse Cardiovascular and Central Nervous System Events Associated with Dietary Supplements Containing Ephedra Alkaloids, *The New England Journal of Medicine,* 343(25):1833, December 21, 2000.

Healthy People 2010: Tracking Healthy People 2010, U.S. Department of Health and Human Services, November 2000.

Heaney, R.P., There Should Be a Dietary Guideline for Calcium, *The American Journal of Clinical Nutrition,* 71(3):658, March 2000.

Heim, D.L., Holcomb, C.A. and Loughin, T.M., Exercise Mitigates the Association of Abdominal Obesity with High-density Lipoprotein Cholesterol in Premenopausal Women: Results from the Third National Health and Nutrition Examination Survey, *Journal of the American Dietetics Association,* 100(11):1347, November 2000.

Hill, J.O. and John C. Peters. Environmental Contributions to the Obesity Epidemic, *Science,* 280:1371, 1998.

Hoffman-Goetz, L., Influenece of Physical Activity and Exercise on Innate Immunity, *Nutrition Reviews,* 56(1):S126, January 1998.

Hogbin, M.B. and Hess, M.A., Public Confusion Over Food Portions and Servings, *Journal of the American Dietetics Association,* 99(10): 1209, October 1999.

Hu, F.B., Stampfer, M.J., Colditz, G.A., et al, Physical Activity and Risk of Stroke in Women, *Journal of the American Medical Association,* 283(22):2961, June 14, 2000.

Hurley, J.S., *Wellness Nutrition & Health,* The Dushkin Publishing Group, Guilford, CT, 1992.

Ikeda, J. P., Hayes, D., Satter, E., Parham, E.S., Kratina, K., Woolsey, M., Lowey, M. and Tribole, E., A Commentary on the New Obesity Guidelines from NIH, *Journal of the American Dietetics Association,* 99(8):918, August 1999.

Irwin, M. Mayer-Davis, E., Addy, C., et. al, Moderate-intensity Physical Activity and Fasting Insulin Levels in Women: The Cross-cultural Activity Participation Study, *Diabetes Care,* 23(4):449, April 2000.

Jakicic, J.M., Winters, C., Lang, W. and Wing, R.R., Effects of Intermittent Exercise and Use of Home Exercise Equipment on Adherence, Weight Loss, and Fitness in Overweight Women, *Journal of the American Medical Association,* 282:1554, 1999.

Kant, A., Consumption of Energy-dense, Nutrient-poor Foods by Adult Americans: Nutrition and Health Implications, The Third National Health and Examination Survey, 1988–1994, *American Journal of Clinical Nutrition,* 72:929, October 2000.

Kernan, W. N., Viscoli, C.M., Brass, L.M., Broderick, J.P., Brott, T., Feldmann, E., Morgenstern, L.B., Wilterdink, J.L. and Horowitz, R.I., Phenylpropanolamine and the Risk of Hemorrhagic Stroke, *The New England Journal of Medicine,* 343(25): 1826, December 21, 2000.

Klem, M.L., Wing, R.R., McGuire, M.T., Seagle, H.M. and Hill, J.O., A Descriptive Study of Individuals Successful at Long-term Maintenance of Substantial Weight Loss, *American Journal of Clinical Nutrition,* 66(2):239, August 1997.

Kolasal, K.M. , Evidence-based Medicine: What Is It and How Does a Dietitian Use It? *Topics in Clinical Nutrition,* 15(4):19, 2000.

Kretsch, M.J., Fong, A.K.H. and Green, M.W., Behavioral and Body Size Correlates of Energy Intake Underreporting by Obese and Normal-weight Women, *Journal of the American Dietetics Association,* 99(3):300, March 1999.

Lakka, T., Laukkanen, J., Rauramaa, R., et.al, Cardiorespiratory Fitness and the Progression of Carotid Artherosclerosis in Middle-aged Men, *Annals of Internal Medicine,* 134:12, January 2, 2001.

Lee, I-M., Rexrode, K.M., Cook, N.R., Manson, J.E. and Buring, J.E., Physical Activity and Coronary Heart Disease in Women: Is "No Pain, No Gain" Passé?, *Journal of the American Medical Association,* 285(11):1447, March 21, 2001.

Lemmer, J.T., Hurlbut, D.E., Martel, G.F., et. al, Age and Gender Responses to Strength Training and Detraining, *Medicine & Science in Sports & Exercise,* 32(8):1505, 2000.

Levine, J., Baukol, P. and Pavlidis, I., Letter: The Energy Expended in Chewing Gum, *New England Journal of Medicine,* 341(27):2100, December 30, 1999.

Levine, J.A., Eberhardt, N.L. and Jensen, M.D., Role of Nonexercise Activity Thermogenesis in Resistance to Fat Gain in Humans, *Science,* 283:212, January 8, 1999.

Levine, J.A., Schleusner, S.J. and Jensen, M.D., Energy Expenditure of Nonexercise Activity, *American Journal of Clinical Nutrition,* 72(6): 1451, December 2000.

Lindeman, A.K., Quest for Ideal Weight: Costs and Consequences, *Medicine & Science in Sports & Exercise,* 31(8): 1135, 1999.

Lohmann, J. and Kant, A.K., Comparison of Food Groups and Health Claims Appearing in Food Advertisements in 3 Popular Magazine Categories, *Journal of the American Dietetics Association,* 100(11): 1396, November 2000.

Lowe, M., Freidman, M., Mattes, D., et. al, Comparison of Verbal and Pictorial Measures of Hunger During Fasting in Normal Weight and Obese Subjects, *Obesity Research,* 8(8):566, November 2000.

Mahan, L.K. and Escott-Strump, S., *Krause's Food, Nutrition & Diet Therapy,* 9th Ed., W.B. Saunders Company, Philadelphia, 1996.

Mansfield, E., McPherson, R. and Koski, K.G., Diet and Waist-to-Hip Ratio: Important Predictors of Lipoprotein Levels in Sedentary and Active Young Men with No Evidence of Cardiovascular Disease, *Journal of the American Dietetics Association,* 99(11):1373, November 1999.

Manson, J.E., Hu, F.B., Rich-Edwards, J.W., et. al, A Prospective Study of Walking as Compared with Vigorous Exercise in the Prevention of Coronary Heart Disease in Women, *New England Journal of Medicine,* 341(9):650, August 26, 1999.

McCaffree, J., Practice Points: Helping Clients Sort Out and Apply Media Messages, *Journal of the American Dietetics Association,* 101(1):41. January 2001.

McCrory, M.A., Fuss, P.J., McCallum, J.E., Yao, M., Vinken, A.G., Hays, N.P. and Roberts, S. B., Dietary Variety within Food Groups: Association with Energy Intake and Body Fatness in Men and Women, *American Journal of Clinical Nutrition,* 69(3):440, March, 1999.

Messier, S.P., Loeser, R.F., Mitchell, M.N., et. al, Exercise and Weight Loss in Obese Older Adults with Knee Osteoarthritis: A Preliminary Study, *Journal of the American Geriatric Society,* 48(9):1062, September 2000.

Miller, W.C., How Effective Are Traditional Dietary and Exercise Interventions for Weight Loss?, *Medicine & Science in Sports & Exercise,* 31(8):1129. 1999.

Mokdad A.H. et al, The Continuing Epidemic of Obesity in the United States (Research Letter), *Journal of the American Medical Association*, 284:1650, 2000.

Mokdad, A.H., Serdula, M.K., Dietz, W.H., Bowman, B.A. Marks, J.S. and Koplan, J.P., The Spread of the Obesity Epidemic in the United States, *Journal of the American Medical Association*, 282(16): 1519, October 27, 1999.

Moritsugu, K.P., A Report from the Office of the Surgeon General, *Journal of the American Dietetics Association*, 100(9): 1013, September 2000.

Must A., Spadano J., Coakley E.H., Field A.E., Colditz G. and Dietz W.H., The Disease Burden Associated with Overweight and Obesity, *Journal of the American Medical Association*, 282:1529, 1999.

Natow, A.B. and Heslin, J., *Fat Attack Plan*, Pocket Books, New York, 1990.

Natow, A.B. and Heslin, J., *Nutrition for the Prime of Your Life*, McGraw-Hill, New York, 1983.

Nieman, D.C., Henson, D.A., Nehlsen-Cannarella, S.L., Ekkens, M., Utter, A.C., Butterworth, D.E. and Fagoaga, O.R., Influence of Obesity on Immune Function, *Journal of the American Dietetics Association*, 99(3):294, March 1999.

NIH Consensus Development Panel on Physical Activity and Cardiovascular Health, *Journal of the American Medical Association*, 276(3): 241, July 17, 1996.

Pace, B., JAMA Patient Page: Benefits of Physical Activity for the Heart, *Journal of the American Medical Association*, 285(11):1536, March 21, 2001.

Patterson, R.E., Satia, J.A., Kristal, A.R., Neuhouser, M.L. and Drewnowski, A., Is There a Consumer Backlash against the Diet and Health Message?, *Journal of the American Dietetics Association*, 101(1): 37, January 2001.

Peppard, P.S., Young, T., Palta, M., Dempsey, J., and Skatrud, J., Longitudinal Study of Moderate Weight Change and Sleep-Disordered Breathing, *Journal of the American Medical Association*, 284(23):3015, December 20, 2000.

Prentice, W.E., *Fitness and Wellness for Life*, 6th Ed., McGraw-Hill, New York, 1999.

Ratzin Jackson, C. G., *Nutrition for the Recreational Athlete,* CRC Press, Boca Raton, 1995.

Ravussin, E., Danford, E., Beyond Sloth—Physical Activity and Weight Gain, *Science,* 283:184, January 8, 1999.

Rebro, S.M., Patterson, R.E., Kristal, A.R. and Cheney, C.L., The Effect of Keeping Food Records on Eating Patterns, *Journal of the American Dietetics Association,* 98(10):1163, October 1998.

Reeves, R.S., McPherson, S., Nichaman, M.Z., et al., Nutrient Intake of Obese Female Binge Eaters, *Journal of the American Dietetic Association,* 101(2):209, February 2001.

Rolls, B.J., Bell, E.A. and Thorwart, M.L., Water Incorporated into a Food but Not Served with a Food Decreases Energy Intake in Lean Women, *American Journal of Clinical Nutrition,* 70(4):448, October 1999.

Rolls, B.J., Bell, E.A. and Waugh, B., Increasing the Volume of a Food by Incorporating Air Affects Satiety in Men, *American Journal of Clinical Nutrition,* 72:361, August 2000.

Ross, C.E. and Hayes, D., Exercise and Psychologic Well-being in the Community, *American Journal of Epidemiology,* 127:762, 1988.

Rowe, S.B., Food for Thought: An In-Depth Look at How the Media Report Nutrition, Food Safety, and Health, *American Medical Writers Association Journal,* 15(4):5, Fall 2000.

Saltzman, E., Dallal, G.E. and Roberts, S.B., Effect of High-fat and Low-fat Diets on Voluntary Energy Intake and Substrate Oxidation; Studies in Identical Twins Consuming Diets Matched for Energy Density, Fiber and Palatability, *American Journal of Clincial Nutrition,* 66(6):1332, December 1997.

Sandler, R.S., Who Wants a Healthful Breakfast?, *New England Journal of Medicine,* 330(16):1162, April 1994.

Schaumberg, D.A., Glynn, R.J., Christen, W.G., Hankinson, S.E. and Hennekens, C.H., Relations of Body Fat Distribution and Height with Cataract in Men, *American Journal of Clinical Nutrition,* 72(6):1495, December 2000.

Shepard, T., Weil, K., Sharp, T., et al., Occasional Physical Inactivity Combined with a High-fat Diet May Be Important in the Development and Maintenance of Obesity in Human Subjects, *American Journal of Clinical Nutrition,* 73: 703, April 2001.

Sparti, A., Milon, H., Di Vetta, V., Schneiter, P., Tappy, L., Jequier, E. and Schutz, Y., Effects of Diets High or Low in Unavailable and Slowly Digestible Carbohydrates on the Pattern of 24-H Substrate Oxidation and Feelings of Hunger in Humans, *American Journal of Clinical Nutrition,* 72(6):1461, December 2000.

Stefanick, M.I., Mackey, S., Sheehan, M., et. al, Effect of Diet and Exercise in Men and Postmenopausal Women with Low Levels of HDL Cholesterol and High Levels of LDL Cholesterol, *New England Journal of Medicine,* 339:12, July 2, 1998.

Steinberg, D., and Gotto, A.M., Preventing Coronary Artery Disease by Lowering Cholesterol Levels, *Journal of the American Medical Association,* 282(21):2043, December 1, 1999.

Stevens, J., Cai, J., Pamuk, E.R., Williamson, D.F., Thun, M.J. and Wood, J.L., The Effect of Age on the Association between Body-Mass Index and Mortality, *The New England Journal of Medicine,* 338(1):1, January 1, 1998.

Stewart, G.W., *Active Living,* Human Kinetics, Champaign, IL, 1995.

Tapsell, L.C., Brenninger, V. and Barnard, J., Applying Conversation Analysis to Foster Accurate Reporting in the Diet History Interview, *Journal of the American Dietetics Association,* 100(7):818, July 2000.

Tiwary, C. M., Ward, J. A. and Jackson, B. A., Effect of Pectin on Satiety in Healthy U.S. Army Adults, *Journal of the American College of Nutrition,* 16 (5):423, 1997.

Van Way III, C.W., *Nutrition Secrets,* Hanley & Belfus, Inc., Philadelphia, 1999.

Vuckovic, N., Ritenbaugh, C., Douglas, T. and Tobar, M., A Qualitative Study of Participants' Experiences with Dietary Assessment, *Journal of the American Dietetics Association,* 100(9):1023, September 2000.

Verloop, J., et. al, Physical Activity and Breast Cancer Risk in Women Aged 20–54 Years, *Journal of the National Cancer Institute,* 92:128, 2000.

Vogler, G.P., Influences of Genes and Shared Family Environment on Adult Body Mass Index Assessed by a Comprehensive Path Model in an Adoption Study," *International Journal of Obesity,* 19:40, 1995.

Way, W.L., Food-related Behaviors on Prime-time Television, *Journal of Nutrition Education,* 15(3):105, 1983.

Wee, C.C., McCarthy, E.P., Davis, R.B. and Phillips, R.S., Physician Counseling about Exercise, *Journal of the American Medical Association,* 282(16):1583, October 27, 1999.

Wei, M., Kampert, J.B., Barlow, C.E., Nichaman, M.Z., Gibbons, L.W., Paffenbenbarger, R.S. and Blair, S.N., Relationship between Low Cardiorespiratory Fitness and Mortality in Normal-weight, Overweight, and Obese Men, *Journal of the American Medical Association,* 282(16):1547, October 27, 1999.

Wickelgren, I. and Taubes, G., Obesity: How Big a Problem, *Science* 280(1988):1366,

Willett, W.C., Guidelines for Healthy Weight, *The New England Journal of Medicine,* 341 (6): 427, August 5, 1999.

Yanovski, J.A., Yanovski, S.Z., Sovik, S.N., Nguyen, T.T., O'Neil, P.M. and Sebring, N.G., A Prospective Study of Holiday Weight Gain, *New England Journal of Medicine,* 342(12):861, March 23, 2000.

Yaroch, A.L., Resnicow, K., Davis, M., Davis, A., Smith, M. and Khan, L.K., Development of a Modified Picture-sort Food Frequency Questionnaire Administered to Low-income, Overweight, African-American Adolescent Girls, *Journal of the American Dietetics Association,* 100(9):1050, September 2000.

Young, L. and Nestle, M., Portion Sizes in Dietary Assessment: Issues and Policy Implications, *Nutrition Reviews,* 53(6):149, June 1995.

Young, L. and Nestle, M., Variation in Perceptions of a "Medium" Food Portion: Implications for Dietary Practice, *Journal of the American Dietetics Association,* 98(4):458, April 1998.

Zemel, M.B., Shi, H, Greer, B., Dirienzo, D. and Zemel, P.C., Regulation of Adiposity by Dietary Calcium, *Federation of American Societies for Experimental Biology,* 14(9):1132, June 2000.

Zorrilla, G., Hunger and Satiety, *Journal of the American Dietetics Association,* 98(10):1111, October 1998.

Recipe Index

General Index

(t = table)

About the Authors

Annette B. Natow, Ph.D., R.D., and Jo-Ann Heslin, M.A., R.D., are the authors of twenty-seven books on nutrition, including two college textbooks. Both are former faculty members of Adelphi University and the State University of New York, Downtown Medical Center. They are the editors of the *Journal of Nutrition for the Elderly,* and serve as editorial board members for *American Baby* and *Vitality* magazines, and *Environmental Nutrition Newsletter.*

For more information on *Get Skinny the Smart Way* go to smartskinny.com

For information about other books by Annette B. Natow and Jo-Ann Heslin go to www.thenutritionexperts.com